LOW-FODMAP DIET *Cookbook* FOR BEGINNERS

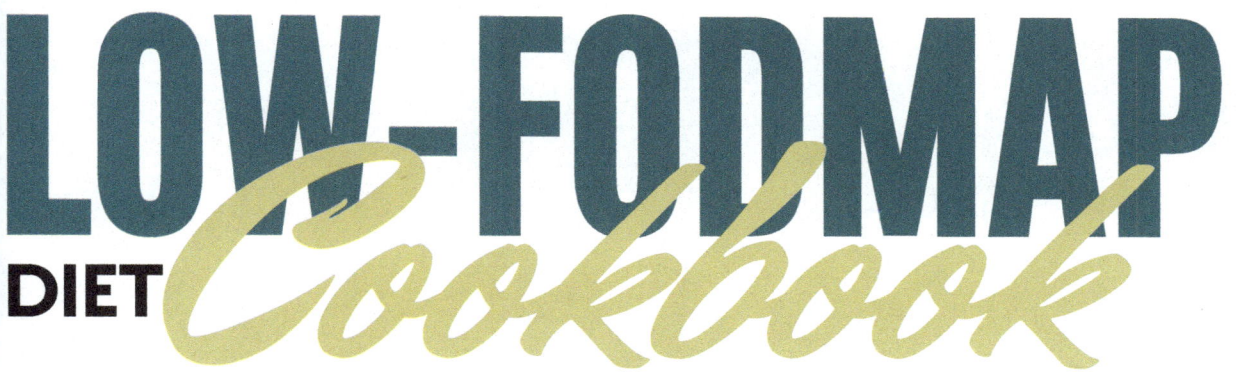

Gut Health Made Delicious with **100+ EASY RECIPES** for IBS and Digestive Relief

28-Days Meal Plan and Shopping List

Sheryl Thompson

Copyright 2025 Sheryl Thompson - All rights reserved.

This publication is subject to copyright protection. This publication is intended for personal use only. Without the author or publisher's permission, it is prohibited to modify, distribute, sell, use, quote, or paraphrase any portion of this book or its content.

No legal liability or culpability will be assigned to the publisher or author for any damages, reparation, or monetary loss that may result from the information contained within this book. Either directly or indirectly. You are accountable for your own decisions, actions, and outcomes.

Disclaimer Notice:

Please be advised that the information in this document is intended solely for educational and entertainment purposes. Every effort has been made to ensure that the information provided is complete, accurate, and reliable. There are no warranties, either expressed or implied. Readers recognize that the author is not providing legal, financial, medical, or professional advice. The content of this book has been compiled from a variety of sources. It is recommended that you seek the advice of a licensed professional prior to implementing any of the techniques described in this book.

TABLE OF CONTENTS

Rice Flour Crepes and Raspberries	19
Tortilla Baked Eggs	20
Banana Muffins	20
Tropical Millet Porridge	21
Grilled Zucchini with Poached Eggs	21
Maple Granola	22
Pumpkin Coconut Milk Smoothie	22

Chapter 1: Overview of Gut Health and Common Issues 6

What Is the Low-FODMAP Diet?	7
Why Does the Low-FODMAP Diet Work?	8
Low, Moderate and High FODMAPs Table	9
The Three Phases of the Low-FODMAP Diet	14

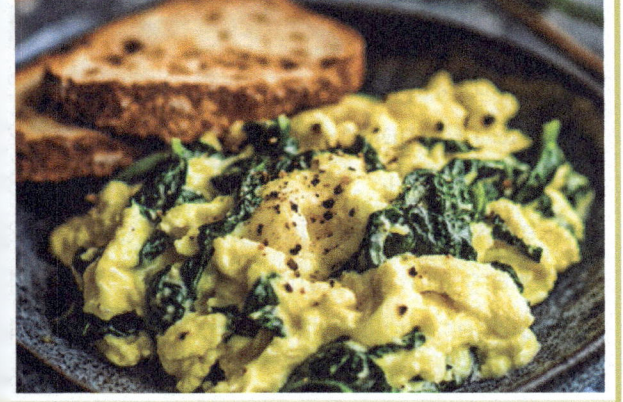

Chapter 3: The Three S's: Salads, Soups, and Sides 23

Grapefruit Prawn Salad	24
Maple Glazed Baby Carrots	25
Caprese Salad	25
Zucchini and Bell Pepper Salad	26
Spinach-Orange Salad with Nuts	26
Parmesan and Thyme Parsnips	27
Vegetable & Chickpea Soup	27
Spinach Salad with Strawberries	28
Beans and Carrots in Vinaigrett	28
Chicken Ramen Noodle Soup	29
Carrot and Parsnip Puree	30
Quinoa Tabbouleh with Cucumber	30
Saltbush Dukkah	31
Sweet Potato with Rosemary	31
Nicoise Salad with Tuna	32
Spaghetti Squash with Olive Oil	32

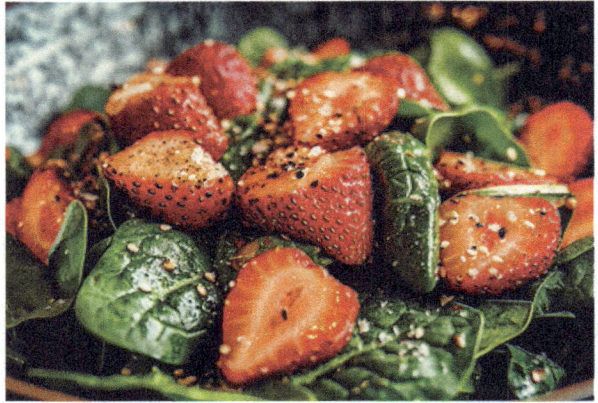

Chapter 2: Rise and Shine Breakfasts 15

Zucchini Sweet Potato Fritters	16
Scrambled Eggs with Spinach	16
Sweet Potato and Kale Hash	17
Quinoa Porridge with Kiwi	17
Fried Plantain and Mint Salad	18
Cinnamon Coconut Rice Porridge	18
Granola with Almond Milk	19

Chapter 4: Flavor-Packed Main Dishes — 33

Quinoa-Stuffed Bell Peppers	34
Garlic-Infused Shrimp Skillet	35
Oven-Baked Cod with Lemon	35
Beef Stir-Fry with Broccoli	36
Sweet Potato Crusted Chops	36
Sesame Chicken and Vegetable Bowl	37
Herb-Grilled Chicken Breast	38
Zucchini Noodles with Pesto Sauce	38
Thai Basil Chicken Stir-Fry	39
Moroccan Spiced Fish Tagine	39
Grilled Pork with Herbs	40
Baked Tilapia with Dill Sauce	40
Eggplant Ratatouille	41
Lemon and Herb Turkey Patties	41
Chicken Coconut Curry	42
Tomato Basil Spaghetti Squash	42
Roasted Chicken Drumsticks	43
Beef Kebabs with Veggies	43
Pan-Seared Scallops with Lemon	44
BBQ-Style Chicken Thighs	44

Chapter 5: Green and Clean Vegetarian & Vegan Dishes — 45

Chickpea-Free Hummus Wrap	46
Vegan Shepherd's Pie	46
Coconut Curry Lentil Soup	47
Eggplant and Tomato Casserole	47
Roasted Vegetable Buddha Bowl	48
Lentil and Spinach Curry	48
Tofu Stir-Fry with Green Beans	49
Zucchini Lasagna with Ricotta	49
Gluten-Free Veggie Pizza	50
Sweet Potato Patties	50

Chapter 6: Quick Fueling Snacks — 51

Roasted Chickpeas	52
Roasted Pumpkin Seeds	52
Raspberry Chia Jam	53
Baked Kale Chips with Lemon Zest	53
Crackers with Cucumber Spread	54
Cucumber Sticks with Hummus	54
Sweet Potato Chips	55
Mini Zucchini Fritters	55
Banana Energy Balls	56
Baked Polenta Squares	56

Chapter 7: Wholesome Dessert Creations — 57

Strawberry and Kiwi Sorbet	58
Raspberry Coconut Milk Popsicles	58
Kiwi and Strawberry Tartlets	59
Carrot Cake with Almond Frosting	59

Coconut Rice Pudding with Orange	60
Raspberry and Almond Crumble	60
Rice Pudding	61
Coconut Macaroons	61
Wattleseed Self-Saucing Pudding	62
Stewed Rhubarb with Ginger	63
Refreshing Mixed Fruit Salad	63
Lemon Myrtle Sorbet	64
Zucchini Chocolate Cake	64

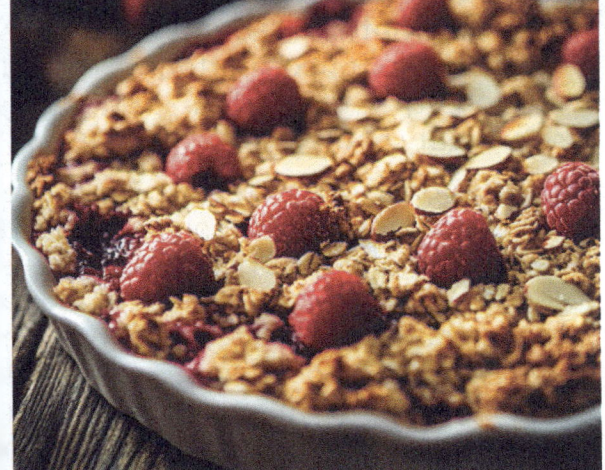

Chapter 8: Bonus: Homemade Sauces and Dressings — 65

Homemade Tomato Sauce	66
Homemade Tahini	66
Homemade Vegetable Broth	67
Fresh Herb Pesto Sauce	67
Sweet Mustard Sauce	68
Roasted Bell Pepper Sauce	68
Almond Butter Sauce	68
Garlic-Infused Mayo Dipping Sauce	69
Ginger and Soy Marinade	69
Lemon Vinaigrette	69
Homemade Chicken Stock	70
Garlic-Infused Olive Oil	70

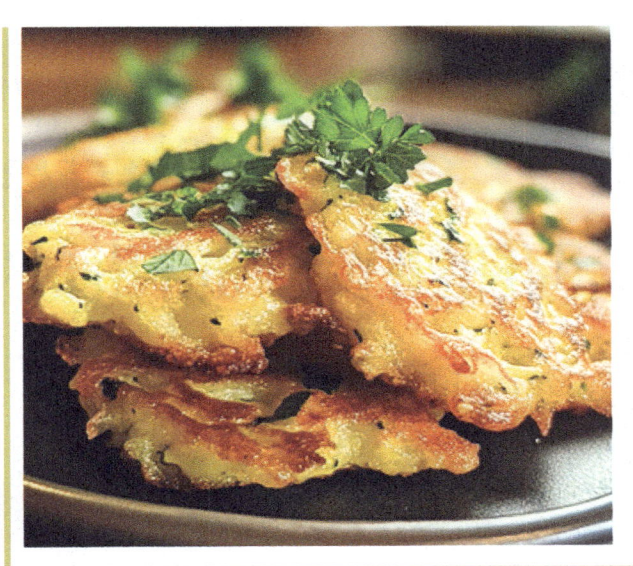

Chapter 9: 28-Day Meal Plan and Shopping List — 71

Meal Plan for Elimination Week 1	72
Shopping List for Week 1	73
Meal Plan for Week 2	74
Shopping List for Week 2	75
Meal Plan for Week 3	76
Shopping List for Week 3	77
Meal Plan for Week 4	78
Shopping List for Week 4	79
Transitioning Out of the Diet Phase	80

Conclusion: A Big Step Toward Improving Your Health — 81

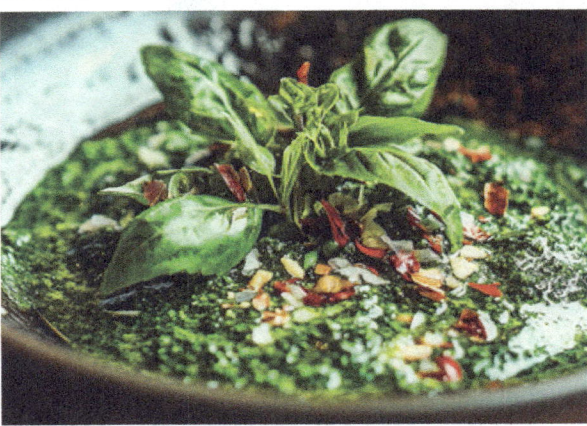

"To eat is a necessity, but to eat intelligently is an art." — François de la Rochefoucauld

Chapter 1:
OVERVIEW OF GUT HEALTH AND COMMON ISSUES

Gut health is foundational to how we feel every day, yet many of us don't give it much thought until something goes wrong. Maybe it's bloating after a meal, discomfort that seems to come out of nowhere, or more persistent symptoms like diarrhea or constipation.

These types of digestive issues are often linked to conditions like Irritable Bowel Syndrome (IBS), which affects **1 in 7 people** worldwide.

Irritable Bowel Syndrome (IBS) is a common digestive condition that affects millions of people, yet it often goes undiagnosed or misdiagnosed for years. IBS is a functional gastrointestinal disorder, which means that while there may not be any visible damage to the intestines, the gut isn't working as it should.

The symptoms of IBS can vary, but they typically include bloating, cramping, diarrhea, constipation, or a combination of all four. For many, these symptoms can be both physically uncomfortable and emotionally distressing, affecting their quality of life.

And unfortunately, for many, these problems are hard to solve because they're not always about one simple cause. What might work for one person could be a trigger for someone else. But the good news? You don't have to just "live with it."

By understanding what's going on inside your gut, you can take control of your digestive health and feel better overall.

THIS IS WHERE THE LOW-FODMAP DIET CAN MAKE A REAL DIFFERENCE!

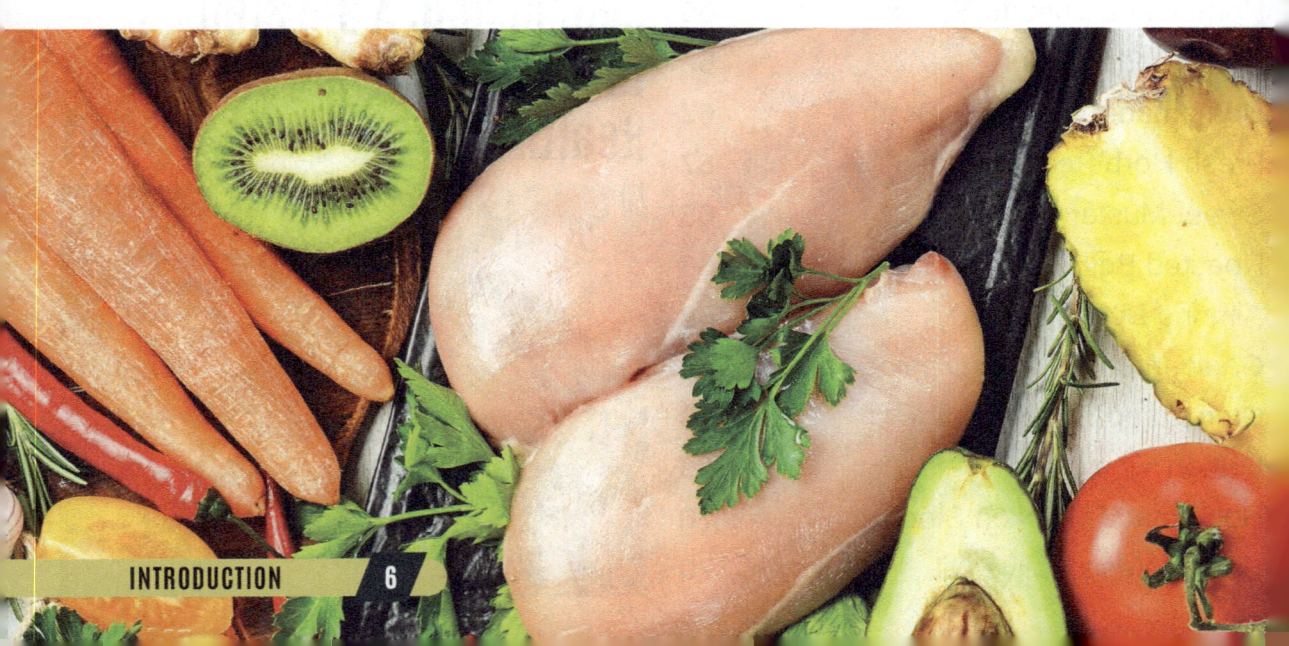

INTRODUCTION

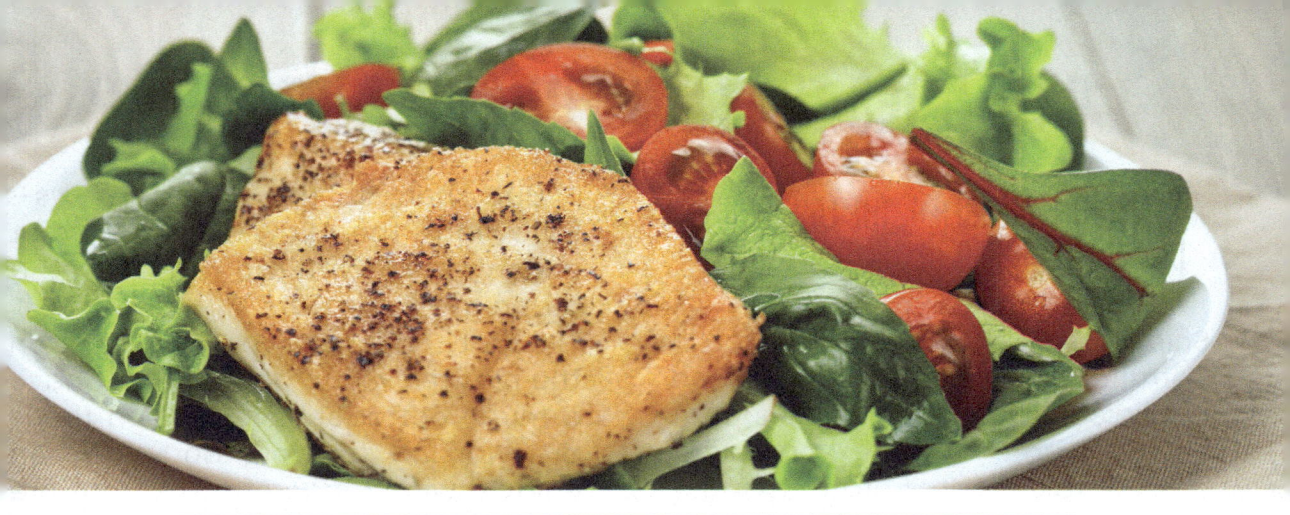

WHAT IS THE LOW-FODMAP DIET?

The Low-FODMAP diet is a structured way of eating that focuses on identifying foods that might be causing digestive issues by eliminating high-FODMAP foods, then reintroducing them gradually to figure out which ones are triggers.

The goal isn't to restrict foods forever; rather, it's to pinpoint the foods that your digestive system might not tolerate well. Developed by researchers at **Monash University**, this diet has gained recognition as one of the most effective ways to manage symptoms of IBS and other gut issues.

So, what exactly are **FODMAPs**? Let's break it down.

WHAT ARE FODMAPS?

FODMAPs are a group of **carbohydrates** (or sugars) that are poorly absorbed in the small intestine and are easily fermented by bacteria in the gut.

This fermentation can produce gas, leading to bloating, cramping, and other digestive discomforts.

FODMAPs are found in a wide variety of foods, and the trick is identifying which ones cause you trouble. Here's what each letter in FODMAP stands for:

- **F = Fermentable:** Refers to the process by which these carbohydrates are fermented in the gut, creating gas.
- **O = Oligosaccharides:** Found in foods like wheat, onions, and garlic.
- **D = Disaccharides:** Found in dairy products like milk and yogurt (the lactose in these foods is a disaccharide).
- **M = Monosaccharides:** Includes fructose, found in fruits like apples, honey, and high-fructose corn syrup.
- **A = And**
- **P = Polyols:** Sugar alcohols found in foods like stone fruits (e.g., cherries, peaches), certain vegetables, and artificial sweeteners.

For many people, these FODMAPs can trigger digestive symptoms.

The Low-FODMAP diet helps reduce these triggers by eliminating high-FODMAP foods and then reintroducing them slowly to see which ones cause problems.

THIS WAY, YOU CAN STILL ENJOY A WIDE VARIETY OF FOODS WHILE LEARNING HOW TO MANAGE YOUR GUT HEALTH.

INTRODUCTION

WHY DOES THE LOW-FODMAP DIET WORK?

AS MENTIONED EARLIER, THE LOW-FODMAP DIET IS GROUNDED IN SOLID RESEARCH.

Scientists at Monash University in Australia developed the diet based on clinical trials and studies that showed how these particular carbohydrates can irritate the gut and cause uncomfortable symptoms for many people, especially those with conditions like IBS.

When you remove high-FODMAP foods and then reintroduce them, it allows you to pinpoint specific triggers and take a more personalized approach to your diet.

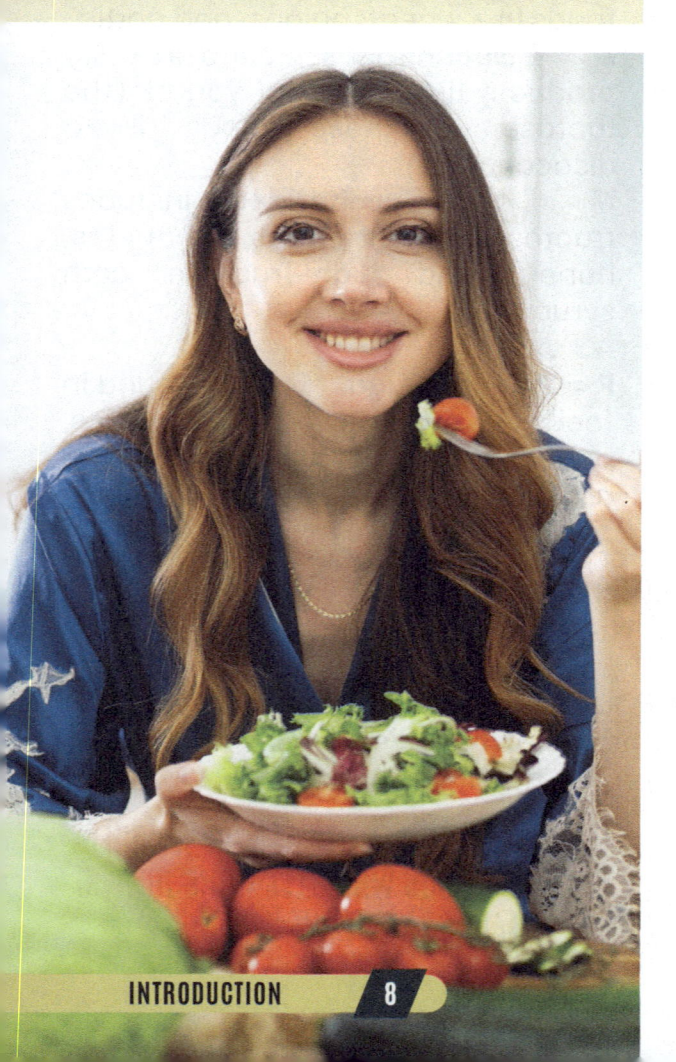

But here's the good news—following the Low-FODMAP diet doesn't mean you'll be stuck eating bland meals forever.

In fact, once you've gone through the reintroduction phase, you'll have a much better sense of which foods are working for you, and you can enjoy a wide range of foods that are still good for your gut.

I'VE WORKED WITH MANY CLIENTS WHO HAVE SEEN INCREDIBLE IMPROVEMENTS IN THEIR GUT HEALTH AFTER ADOPTING THE LOW-FODMAP DIET.

Take Emily, for example, a client of mine who had struggled with bloating, stomach pain, and irregular digestion for years.

She tried every remedy under the sun, from probiotics to cutting out dairy, but nothing really seemed to make a difference.

After starting the Low-FODMAP diet, she began to notice patterns.

She learned that onions, garlic, and certain wheat-based products were causing the bulk of her discomfort.

Once she eliminated those, and reintroduced them slowly, she could finally enjoy a balanced diet without the constant fear of digestive issues.

Practical Tip:

If you're just starting out, try not to feel overwhelmed.

Yes, there's a lot of detail to consider, but the key is to take it one step at a time.

With the right approach, you'll feel empowered to take control of your digestive health.

INTRODUCTION

LOW, MODERATE AND HIGH FODMAPS TABLE

When navigating the Low-FODMAP diet, knowing which foods fall into each category is crucial. This information comes from the **Monash University FODMAP Diet App**, a trusted resource developed by researchers who pioneered the diet.

The app uses a simple traffic light rating system—green for low, amber for moderate, and red for high—to help identify FODMAP levels in foods.

Below is a general guide to help you get started.

Note:
This table includes some everyday foods you may encounter, but remember that individual tolerance to FODMAPs can vary, so it's essential to monitor your body's responses during the elimination and reintroduction phases.

LOW FODMAPS *(Green Light - Safe to Eat)*

BREAD, CEREALS, RICE, and PASTA
- Buckwheat
- Flour (arrowroot, buckwheat, cassava, corn, rice, sorghum)
- Flour, gluten-free, plain
- Gluten-free bread
- Gluten-free pasta
- Millet
- Noodle (rice, soba, vermicelli)
- Oats (rolled or quick; plain with no added sweeteners)
- Pastry puff
- Polenta
- Quinoa
- Rice (white, brown, basmati, glutinous)
- Spelt bread, 100%
- Spelt bread, sourdough

VEGETABLES
- Alfalfa
- Bamboo shoots (raw or canned)
- Beans
- Bell pepper (green)
- Bok choy
- Broccoli (heads only)
- Cabbage (Chinese, red, white)
- Carrots
- Celery (leaves only)
- Chilli (green, red)
- Collard greens
- Corn
- Cucumbers
- Eggplant
- Endive, Fennel
- Ginger
- Kale
- Leek (green leaves only)
- Lettuce (romaine, iceberg, radicchio)
- Olives (black, green)
- Parsnip
- Pea, snow
- Potatoes (white, red, sweet)
- Radish
- Spinach (baby spinach, English)
- Turmeric
- Turnip
- Yam

FRUITS
- Bananas (unripe or slightly yellow)
- Blueberries,
- Cranberries (not dried)
- Dates (Medjool or dried)
- Dragonfruit
- Grapefruit
- Jackfruit (young, canned, drained)
- Kiwi
- Mandarins
- Melon, cantaloupe /rockmelon, peeled, deseeded, raw
- Orange
- Papaya (green or yellow)
- Passion fruit
- Pineapple
- Plantain
- Prickly pear
- Tamarind

MEAT, FISH, AND EGGS
- Bacon (all cuts, plain, cooked)
- Beef (all cuts, plain, cooked)
- Chicken (all cuts, plain, cooked)
- Eggs
- Fish (all varieties, plain)
- Lamb (all cuts, plain, cooked)
- Pork (all cuts, plain, cooked)
- Prawn
- Salmon
- Tuna (fresh or canned in water/oil with no added ingredients)
- Turkey (all cuts, plain, cooked)

DAIRY, SOY & LACTOSE-FREE PRODUCTS
- Almond milk (unsweetened)
- Cheeses (cheddar, parmesan, Swiss, gouda, mozzarella, parmesan, cottage, ricotta)
- Whipped cream, fresh
- Pure cream, regular fat
- Sour cream, regular fat
- Coconut milk (light, canned)
- Lactose-free yogurt (natural, regular fat)
- Coconut yoghurt
- Strawberry yoghurt (lactose-free, regular fat)

INTRODUCTION

LOW FODMAPS (Green Light - Safe to Eat)

PULSES, TOFU, AND NUTS

- Canned lentils (rinsed and drained, max ¼ cup)
- Chestnut
- Macadamia nuts
- Pecan nuts
- Peanut
- Walnut
- Chia seeds
- Hemp seed
- Flaxseed
- Poppy seed
- Pumpkin seeds
- Sunflower seeds
- Sesame seeds
- Firm tofu (plain, not silken)
- Tempeh, plain

BEVERAGES

- Beer (gluten-free)
- Coffee (espresso, instant)
- Red wine
- White vine
- Sparkling water
- (unsweetened)
- Herbal teas (e.g., peppermint, rooibos; avoid chamomile and fennel)
- Tea (green or black)

FATS AND OILS

- Butter (plain, unsalted)
- Ghee (clarified butter)
- Avocado oil
- Coconut oil
- Flaxseed oil
- Olive oil
- (extra-virgin or regular)
- Peanut oil
- Rice bran
- Sesame oil
- Sunflower oil
- Truffle oil
- Vegetable oil

CONDIMENTS

- Celery (leaves only), raw
- Chutney, mango/tomato
- Coconut aminos
- Coconut cream, canned, regular fat
- Curry powder
- Eggplant dip
- Herbs de Provence
- Basil (dried & fresh)
- Bay leaves
- Chives (dried & fresh)
- Coriander/cilantro (dried & fresh)
- Curry leaves (fresh)
- Dill
- Fenugreek
- Lemongrass
- Mint
- Oregano (dried & fresh)
- Parsley (dried & fresh)
- Sage (dried & fresh)
- Thyme (dried & fresh)
- Lemon juice (freshly squeezed)
- Mayonnaise (low-fat, regular fat)
- Paste (miso, shrimp, tahini, tamari, tomato)
- Salsa verde
- Sauce (Worcestershire, BBQ, Chimichurri, Fish, Habanero, Hoisin, Oyster, Satay, Soy, Sriracha, Sweet and sour, tamari, tomato)
- Ketchup (Low-FODMAP varieties, check labels)
- Peanut butter (natural, unsweetened)
- Vinegar (apple cider, rice wine, white, malt, red wine)

SNACKS, BARS, AND COOKIES

- Biscuit/Cookie, plain
- Cake, egg, spelt
- Corn chips, plain
- Plain potato chips (no onion/garlic seasoning)
- Chips, potato straws, salted
- Cracker
- (rice, rye, saltines, wheat, wholemeal)
- Popcorn, plain
- Prawn cracker, cooked
- Pretzels
- Rice cake, plain
- Rusk, wholemeal

CONFECTIONERY AND SUGARS

- Agar agar
- Dark chocolate (in small amounts – max 30g)
- Instant jelly (lime, raspberry, strawberry)
- Jelly grass, canned
- Marshmallow
- Orange blossom water
- Rose water
- Brown sugar
- Coconut sugar
- Sugar, icing/powdered/confectioners
- Sugar, jaggery
- Sugar, palm
- Sugar, raw
- Sugar, white
- Stevia (pure, without added sweeteners)
- Maple syrup, pure
- Rice malt syrup
- Vanilla essence

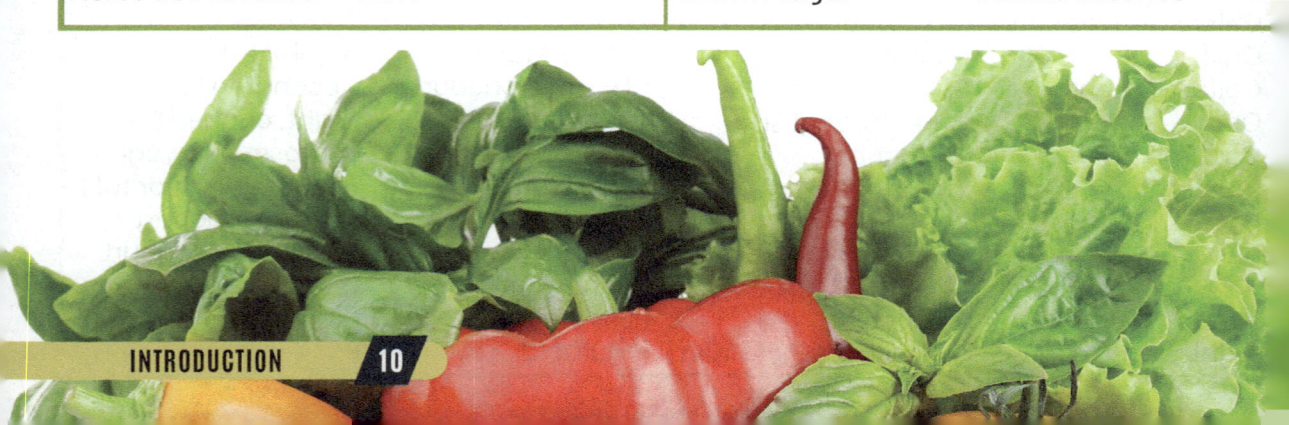

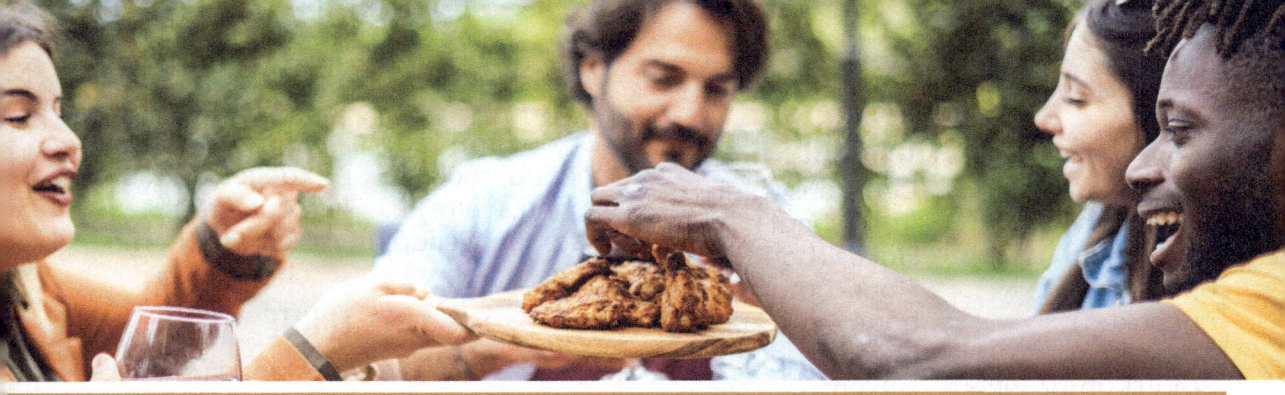

MODERATE FODMAPS *(Amber Light – Consume with Caution)*

BREAD, CEREALS, RICE, AND PASTA

Brown rice flour
Corn flakes cereal
Cooked buckwheat kernels
Cooked egg noodles (wheat-based)
Cooked pearl millet
Fine, organic, gluten-free oatmeal (uncooked)
Gluten-free bread (made with gluten-free wheat starch), sourdough
Gluten-free bread (rice and chia)
Gluten-free bread, high-fiber
Gluten-free bread, mixed grain/multigrain
Millet flour (finger/ragi)
Mixed grain flakes cereal (7-grain mix)
Oat flakes
Pastry, filo, or phyllo dough (cooked)
Puffed or popped rice cereal
Quick oats (uncooked)
Sourdough oat bread

VEGETABLES

Butter lettuce (raw)
Canned whole round tomatoes (with juice)
Raw common tomatoes
Raw okra
Raw zucchini/courgette/baby marrow
Semi-sun-dried tomatoes (drained)
Truss/on-the-vine tomatoes (raw)
Unpeeled butternut squash (raw)

FRUITS

Boysenberries
Cantaloupe/rockmelon
Hass avocado (peeled, pitted, raw)
Pineapple slices (canned in juice, drained)
Raw coconut flesh (from mature fruit)
Raspberries
Strawberries

SNACKS, BARS, AND COOKIES

Chocolate-coated sandwich cookies with cream filling
Plain corn cakes
Shortbread cookies

PULSES, TOFU, AND NUTS

Boiled, hulled red lentils (drained)
Canned chickpeas/Garbanzo beans
Canned, drained red kidney beans
Caraway seeds

BEVERAGES

Black tea (strong)
Chai tea (weak, made with soy milk)
Cranberry juice drink (27% juice)
Chocolate-flavored malted beverage base
Chrysanthemum tea (weak or strong)
Herbal tea (contains chicory root, weak)

FATS AND OILS

None (pure fats and oils are FODMAP-free)

CONDIMENTS

Basil pesto sauce
Balsamic vinegar
Caviar dip
Coconut jam spread
Fruit chutney
(with pear, apple, garlic, and onion)
Quince paste
Soup concentrate

CONFECTIONERY AND SUGARS

Coconut treacle syrup
White chocolate
Milk chocolate

DAIRY, SOY & LACTOSE-FREE PRODUCTS

American cheese (white, pre-wrapped)
Regular-fat vanilla ice cream
Regular-fat vanilla-flavored yogurt
Unsweetened coconut milk (long-life/UHT)

MEAT, FISH, AND EGGS

Cooked German bratwurst sausage

HIGH FODMAPs (Red Light – Avoid in Elimination Phase)

BREAD, CEREALS, RICE, AND PASTA

Almond meal
Bran wheat (processed, unprocessed, uncooked)
Bread Naan/Roti
Bread Kamut, whole meal, sourdough
Bread mixed grain/multigrain, sprouted
Bread (oatmeal, pumpernickel, rye, rye dark, rye light sourdough, spelt ewith honey)
Bread wheat (high fiber, mixed grain/multigrain, raisin/fruit, white, whole meal, wholegrain)
Breakfast cereal (contains dried fruit and nuts, muesli, granola, rice crisps)

Couscous (gluten free, wheat)
Flakes (barley, spelt)
Flour (amaranth, barley, chickpea, chestnut, coconut, einkorn, emmer, Khorasan, lupin, rye, soy, spelt, wheat)
Grain barley (pearl, whole, cooked)
Grain (amaranth, bulgur, farro, spelt, freekeh, rye, wheat germ, whole wheat)
Noodle (dried thin, instant, laksa or wheat)
Pasta, gluten free (red lentil flavor, soy, corn, potato and rice)
Pasta (spelt, wheat)
Porridge (maize)
Semolina
Spelt, flakes

VEGETABLES

Artichoke
Asparagus
Beetroot, raw
Bell pepper (red, orange, yellow)
Bitter melon, raw
Broccoli (stalks only)
Broccolini (heads only)
Brussels sprouts
Cabbage, savoy, raw
Cauliflower white, raw
Celery (stalks only), raw
Chili (jalapeno, ancho, chipotle)
Cuca melon
Garlic, peeled, raw
Garlic shoots, raw
Garlic, black

Gourd (ivy/tindora, frozen)
Kimchi
Leek (white bulb only)
Lotus root, dried
Mushroom black chanterelle, dried
Mushroom, button, raw
Mushroom enoki, raw
Mushroom porcini, dried
Mushroom portobella, raw
Mushroom red pine, raw
Mushroom shitake, (raw, dried)
Mushroom, slippery jack, raw

Onion (Spanish, Vidalia, shallot, spring, white)
Pea, sugar snap (raw)
Peas, green

Pumpkin/squash (delicata, acorn)
Sauerkraut
Tomato (Roma, cherry raw)

FRUITS

Apple
Apple Custard
Apricot
Banana (common, ripe, peeled, raw)
Blackberry raw
Cranberry, dried
Cherries (pitted, raw)
Currants, dried
Figs
Goji berries
Grape (red, green, white, seedless, raw)
Guava (canned in syrup, firm, peeled, raw)
Jackfruit (yellow, freeze, dried, canned)
Longan
Lychee (peeled, pitted, raw)

Mango (dried, peeled, pitted, raw)
Mangosteen (freeze dried)
Melon (honey dew, white skin, peeled, deseeded, raw)
Nectarine (white/yellow, unpeeled, pitted, raw)
Peach
Pear
Persimmon
Pineapple (canned in syrup, slices, drained, dried)
Plum (black diamond)
Pomegranate seeds
Prune/Dried plum
Raisin
Rambutan
Watermelon

MEAT, FISH, AND EGGS

Casserole (canned, French)

DAIRY, SOY & LACTOSE-FREE PRODUCTS

Buttermilk
Cheese with garlic and herb
Condensed milk (from cow, sweetened)
Kefir, plain
Milk (black soy bean, coconut)

Milk (cow, A2, evaporated)
Milk (oat)
Milk soy (sweetened, unsweetened)
Yoghurt (Greek, goat, Indian, natural, soy)
Vanilla custard

CONFECTIONERY AND SUGARS

Fruit Leather
Honey,
Honey (avocado)
Honey (clover)

Syrup (agave, apple, barley malt extract, golden, molasses, sorghum)

FATS AND OILS

None (pure fats and oils are FODMAP-free)

INTRODUCTION 12

HIGH FODMAPs *(Red Light - Avoid in Elimination Phase)*

PULSES, TOFU, AND NUTS

Baked beans
Bean (Adzuki/Red Chori, dried, boiled, drained)
Bean (Navy, dried, boiled, drained)
Bean (black, borlotti, broad, butter, cannellini, haricot, lima, moth, pinto, red kidney, soya, lentil)
Chana Dal
Chickpea
Falafel
Four bean mix (cannellini beans, chickpeas, red kidney beans, lima beans)
Nut (almond, cashew, hazelnut, pine, pistachio)
Pea, Lentil soup
Tofu (soy bean curd), silken
Toor Dal

BEVERAGES

Aloe drink, unflavored
Apple juice (99% reconstituted)
Carob powder
Coconut water
Cola
Cordial, apple and raspberry (50% real juice)
Cordial, orange (25-50% real juice)
Juice of berry fruit blend (99% reconstituted)
Kombucha
Lemonade
Malted beverage base
Orange juice
Rum, dark
Tomato juice
Tea black, strong
Tea chai, strong (cow's milk, low fodmap milk alt., soy milk)
Tea chamomile, (strong, weak)
Tea dandelion, strong
Tea, fennel (strong, weak)
Tea herbal (contains chicory root), strong
Tea oolong, (strong, weak)
Wine (sticky, dessert, fortified)

SNACKS, BARS, AND COOKIES

Bar (energy, apple, berry, fruit, nut, oatmeal, raisins, walnut, peanut butter, granola, oat, honey, muesli, snack)
Biscuit/Cookie chocolate chip, fruit filled, multigrain, with currants/raisins)
Corn cake, sour cream chives
Crispbread, rye
Gingerbread Cake
Rice cake, sour cream chives

CONDIMENTS

Applesauce sauce
Currywurst powder
Dip (hummus, tzatziki)
Ketchup
Garlic powder spice
Marinade (barbeque, Cantonese style)
Onion (pickled in vinegar, drained)
Passata
Pasta sauce (cream-based, tomato based)
Spread (jam, blueberry, mixed berry, marmalade, blackcurrant, vegetable pickles/relish)
Tomato puree
Wasabi paste

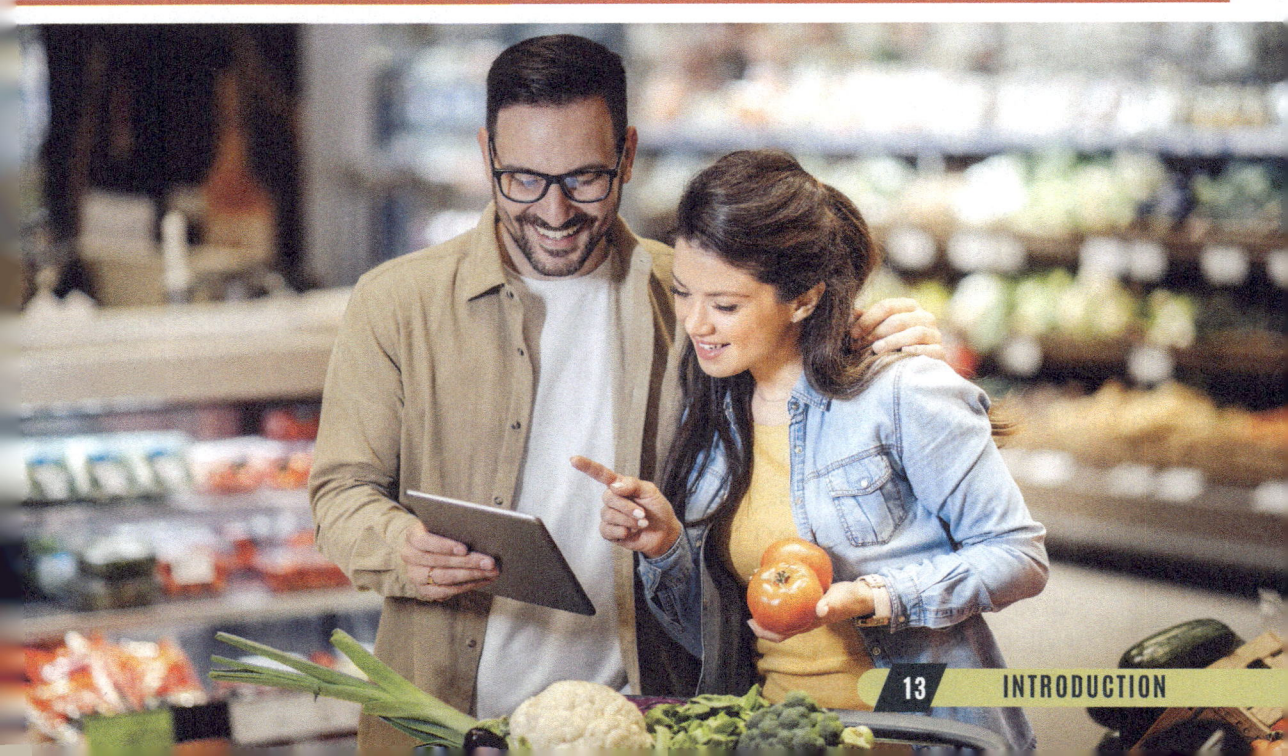

THE THREE PHASES OF THE LOW-FODMAP DIET

The Low-FODMAP diet is divided into three phases. While it may seem a bit complicated at first, it's actually a step-by-step approach that helps you find the foods that work best for your gut.

Phase 1: ELIMINATION

In the first phase of the Low-FODMAP diet, you'll eliminate all high-FODMAP foods for about 4 to 6 weeks. This phase may feel restrictive, but it's necessary to give your gut a break and reduce symptoms like bloating, discomfort, or pain. During this time, you'll focus on eating low-FODMAP foods that are easier on your digestive system. Foods to avoid include:

- Garlic and onions
- Certain dairy products (like milk and soft cheeses)
- High-fructose fruits (such as apples and watermelon)
- Certain legumes (like beans and lentils)

It might feel challenging to cut out these foods at first, but don't worry—there are plenty of delicious alternatives. I'll provide you with some easy and tasty meal ideas to help you get through this phase without feeling deprived.

Phase 2: REINTRODUCTION

After 4 to 6 weeks, you'll begin the reintroduction phase. This is where you'll start reintroducing high-FODMAP foods, one at a time, to see how your body reacts. For example, you might start with a small portion of dairy and check if it causes bloating or discomfort. If it does, you'll know dairy might be a trigger for you. If it doesn't, it's safe to continue eating it. The key is to introduce only one food at a time and track any symptoms. It usually takes most people around 6 to 8 weeks to fully complete this phase, as it's important to give each food time to be assessed. This step helps you figure out what you can tolerate and what you should avoid.

Phase 3: PERSONALIZATION

In the final phase, you'll use everything you've learned from the elimination and reintroduction phases to create a diet that works specifically for you. You'll know which foods are safe to eat, which ones you need to limit, and which ones to avoid. This phase helps you create a long-term, sustainable eating plan that keeps your digestive health in mind while allowing you to enjoy the foods that work best for your body.

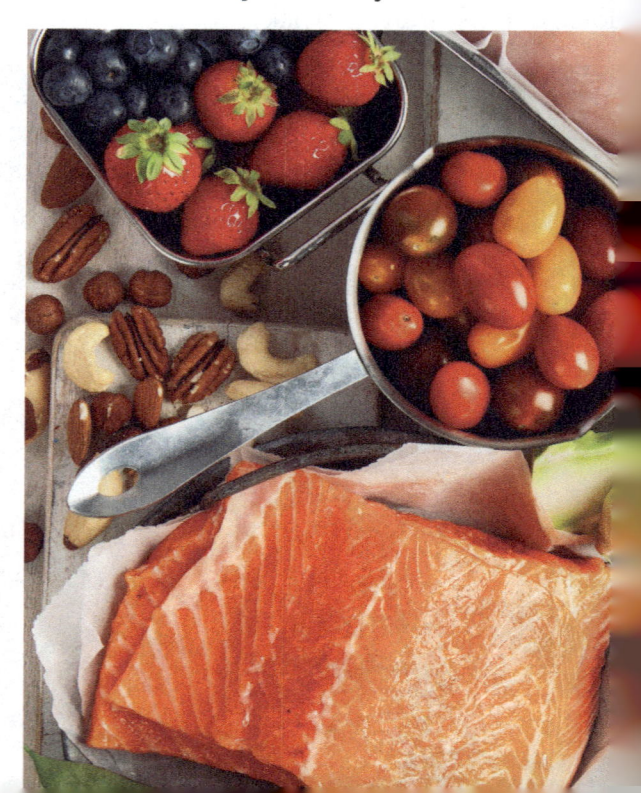

Chapter 2: Rise and Shine
BREAKFASTS

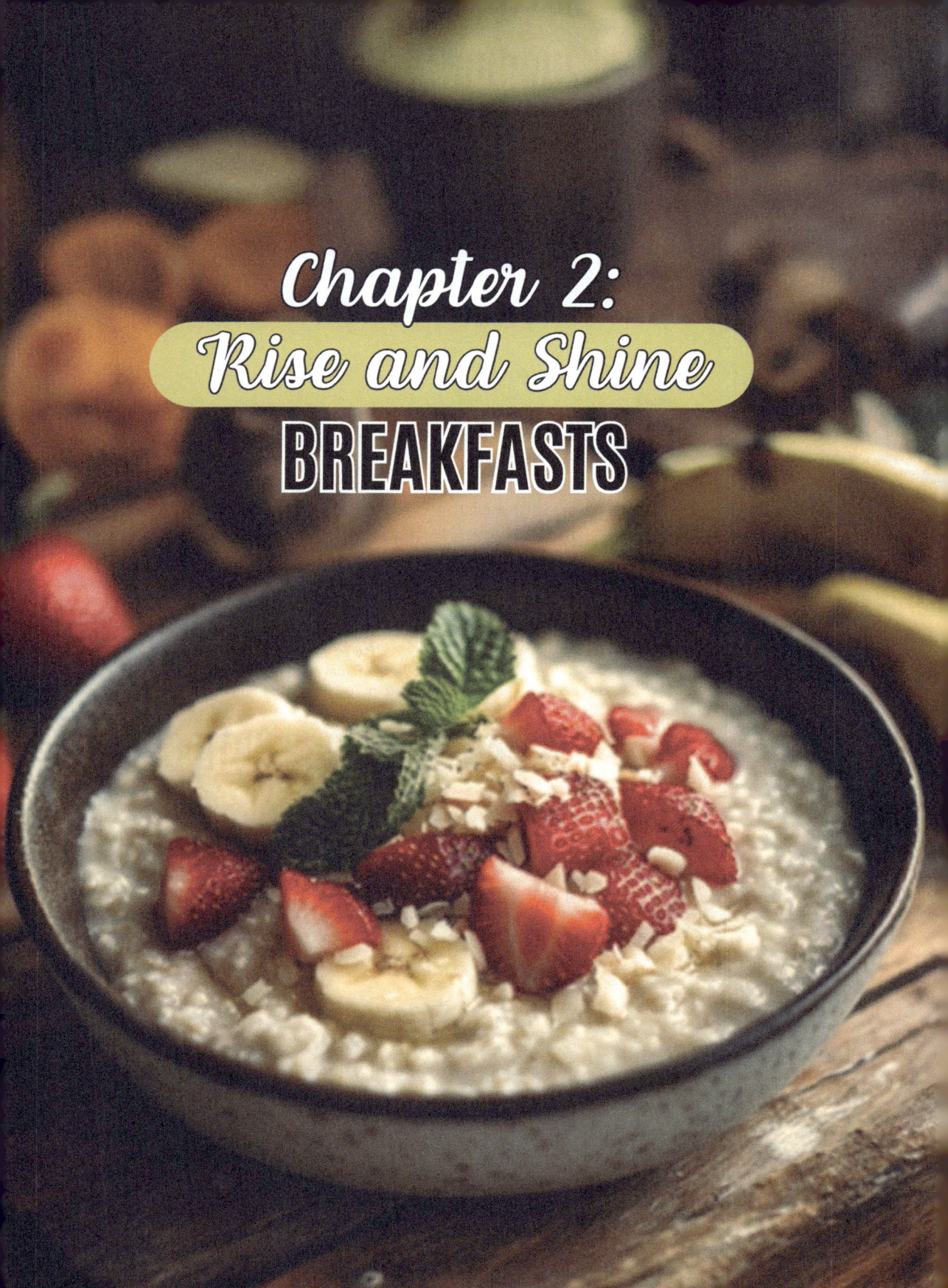

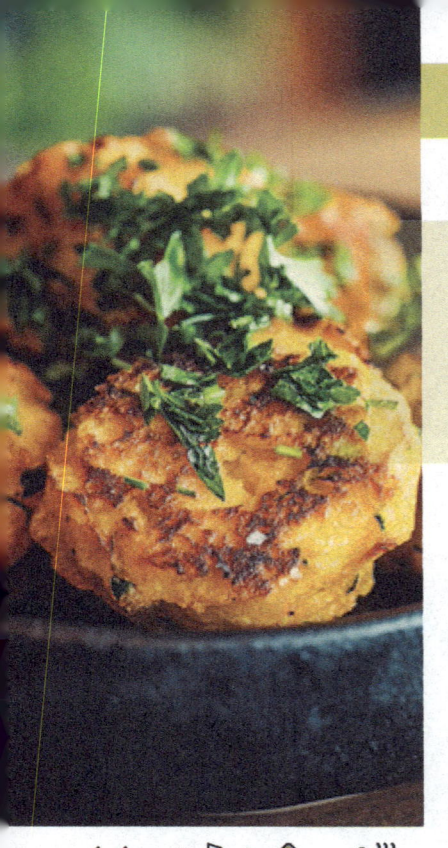

ZUCCHINI SWEET POTATO FRITTERS

Ingredients:

- 1 cup/150g grated zucchini (drain excess moisture with a towel)
- 1 cup/150g grated sweet potato
- 2 large eggs
- 2 tbsps./30g gluten-free flour
- 1 tbsp. chopped fresh parsley
- 2 tsps. olive oil
- Salt and pepper to taste

Instructions:

1. Combine the grated zucchini, sweet potato, parsley, eggs, gluten-free flour, salt, and pepper in a mixing bowl. Mix well to form a batter.
2. Heat olive oil in a non-stick pan set to medium heat. Scoop a spoonful of the mixture into the pan, pressing lightly to form a fritter shape.
3. Cook for 3–4 minutes on each side or until golden brown and cooked through. Repeat until all the batter is used. Serve warm.

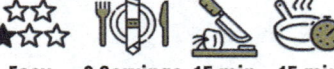

Per serving:
Calories: 260kcal | Fat: 8g | Carbs: 25g | Protein: 7g | Fiber: 4g | Sugar: 5g

Easy | 2 Servings | 15 min | 15 min

Easy | 2 Servings | 5 min | 5 min

SCRAMBLED EGGS WITH SPINACH

Ingredients:

- 4 large eggs
- ½ cup/30g fresh spinach, chopped
- ¼ cup/60ml lactose-free milk
- 1 tbsp. olive oil
- Salt and pepper to taste

Instructions:

1. In your bowl, whisk together eggs, lactose-free milk, salt, and pepper.
2. Heat olive oil in a non-stick skillet set to medium heat.
3. Add spinach and sauté for 1–2 minutes until wilted.
4. Drizzle the egg mixture into the skillet then cook gently, stirring continuously, until soft and creamy.
5. Serve immediately.

Per serving:
Calories: 230kcal | Fat: 12g | Carbs: 3g | Protein: 13g | Fiber: 1g | Sugar: 1g

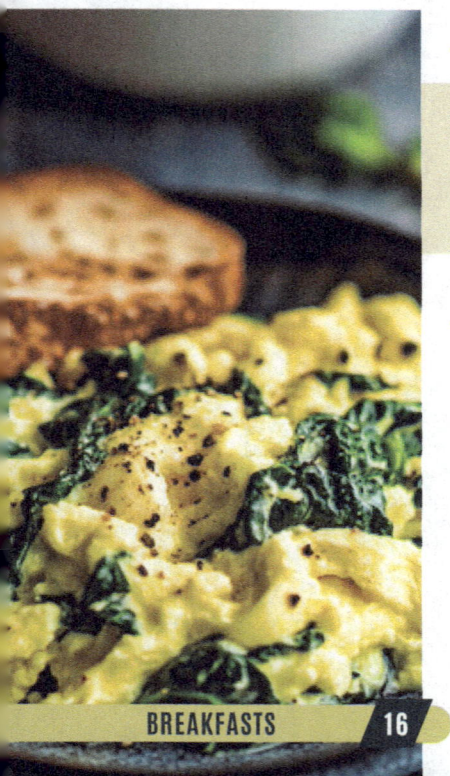

BREAKFASTS

SWEET POTATO AND KALE HASH

Ingredients:

- 1 medium sweet potato, peeled and diced
- 1 cup/67g fresh kale, chopped
- 2 tbsps. olive oil
- ¼ tsp. paprika
- 2 large eggs (optional for protein boost)
- Salt and pepper to taste

Instructions:

1. Heat 1 tbsp. olive oil in a skillet that is set to medium heat. Add diced sweet potatoes and cook for 10 minutes, stirring occasionally, until softened.
2. Add kale and the remaining olive oil. Sauté for 5 minutes until the kale wilts.
3. Season with paprika, salt, and pepper.
4. If adding eggs, make small wells in the mixture and crack the eggs in. Cover and cook for 3–5 minutes until the eggs are set.
5. Serve immediately.

Per serving:
Calories: 250kcal | Fat: 10g | Carbs: 25g | Protein: 4g | Fiber: 4g | Sugar: 5g

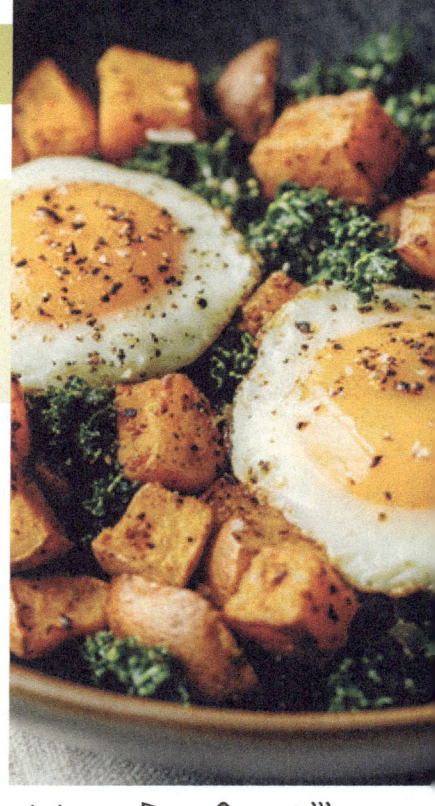

Medium | 2 Servings | 10 min | 20 min

QUINOA PORRIDGE WITH KIWI

Easy | 2 Servings | 5 min | 15 min

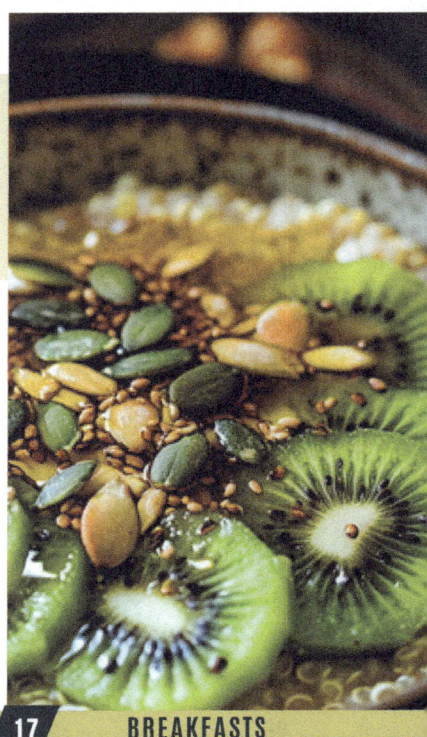

Ingredients:

- ½ cup/90g quinoa, rinsed
- 1 cup/240ml water
- ½ cup/120ml almond milk (unsweetened)
- 1 tsp./5ml pure maple syrup
- 1 medium kiwi, peeled and sliced
- 1 tbsp. pumpkin seeds

Instructions:

1. In a saucepan, bring quinoa and water to a boil. Reduce heat to low, cover, then simmer for 12–15 minutes until water is absorbed.
2. Stir in almond milk and maple syrup. Cook for extra 2–3 minutes until creamy.
3. Divide porridge into bowls and top with kiwi slices and pumpkin seeds. Serve warm.

Per serving:
Calories: 250kcal | Fat: 5g | Carbs: 32g | Protein: 6g | Fiber: 4g | Sugar: 6g

BREAKFASTS

FRIED PLANTAIN AND MINT SALAD

Ingredients:

- 2 ripe plantains, peeled and sliced
- 1 tbsp. olive oil
- 2 tbsps. fresh mint, chopped
- 1 tbsp./15ml lime juice
- Salt to taste

Instructions:

1. Heat olive oil in a skillet set to medium heat.
2. Add plantain slices and fry for 2–3 minutes per side, until golden brown.
3. Remove from heat and place on a paper towel to drain excess oil.
4. In your bowl, toss the fried plantains with chopped mint and lime juice.
5. Season using salt to taste and serve immediately.

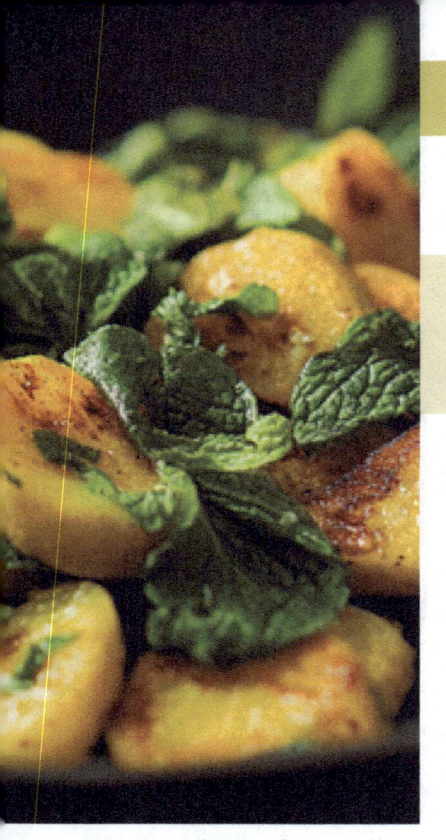

Easy | 2 Servings | 10 min | 5 min

Per serving:
Calories: 300kcal | Fat: 14g | Carbs: 35g | Protein: 2g | Fiber: 4g | Sugar: 12g

---

Easy | 2 Servings | 5 min | 15 min

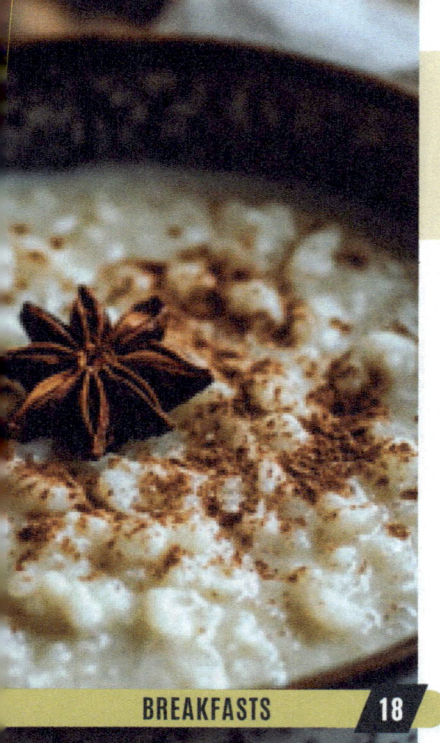

CINNAMON COCONUT RICE PORRIDGE

Ingredients:

- ½ cup/85g jasmine rice
- 1 cup/240ml coconut milk (unsweetened)
- ½ cup/120ml water
- ¼ tsp. cinnamon
- 1 tsp./5ml maple syrup (optional)

Instructions:

1. In a saucepan, bring jasmine rice, coconut milk, and water to a boil.
2. Reduce heat to low and cover. Simmer for 12–15 minutes, until the rice is tender and the mixture thickens.
3. Stir in cinnamon and maple syrup (if using).
4. Serve the porridge warm, and top with additional cinnamon if desired.

Per serving:
Calories: 300kcal | Fat: 14g | Carbs: 30g | Protein: 3g | Fiber: 2g | Sugar: 6g

BREAKFASTS

GRANOLA WITH ALMOND MILK

Ingredients:

- 1 cup/90g gluten-free rolled oats
- 10 pcs/12g raw almonds, chopped
- ¼ cup/30g pumpkin seeds
- 1 tbsp./15ml maple syrup
- 1 tbsp. coconut oil, melted
- ½ cup/120ml unsweetened almond milk

Instructions:

1. Preheat the oven to 350°F/180°C.
2. In your bowl, combine oats, chopped almonds, and pumpkin seeds.
3. Drizzle with melted coconut oil and maple syrup. Mix until the dry ingredients are evenly coated.
4. Apply the mixture on a baking sheet in a single layer and bake for 15–20 minutes, stirring halfway through, until golden brown.
5. Let the granola cool before serving with almond milk.

Per serving:
Calories: 300kcal | Fat: 16g | Carbs: 22g | Protein: 7g | Fiber: 4g | Sugar: 6g

Medium | 2 Servings | 5 min | 20 min

RICE FLOUR CREPES AND RASPBERRIES

Ingredients:

- ½ cup/60g rice flour
- ½ cup/120ml lactose-free milk
- 2 large eggs
- 1 tbsp. olive oil
- ½ cup/60g fresh raspberries
- 1 tbsp./15ml maple syrup (optional)

Instructions:

1. In your bowl, whisk together rice flour, lactose-free milk, eggs, and olive oil until smooth.
2. Heat a non-stick skillet set to medium heat and lightly grease with olive oil.
3. Pour a small amount of batter into the pan, swirling to form a thin crepe.
4. Cook for 1–2 minutes per side, until golden brown.
5. Repeat with the remaining batter. Serve crepes topped with fresh raspberries and a drizzle of maple syrup.

Per serving:
Calories: 280kcal | Fat: 9g | Carbs: 30g | Protein: 6g | Fiber: 4g | Sugar: 7g

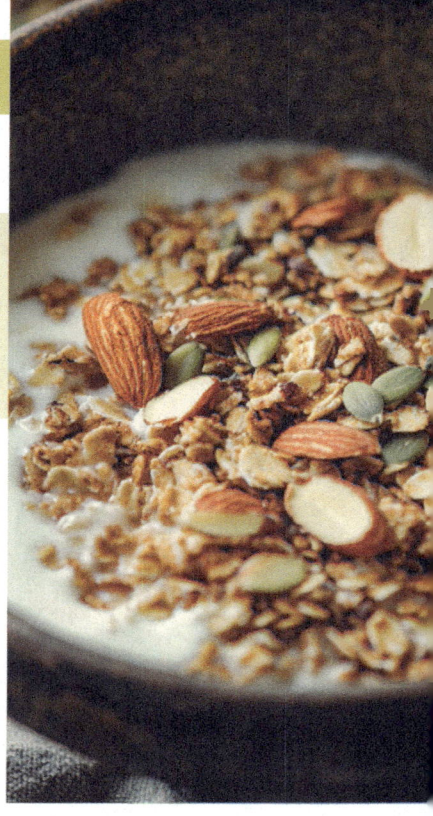

Easy | 2 Servings | 10 min | 10 min

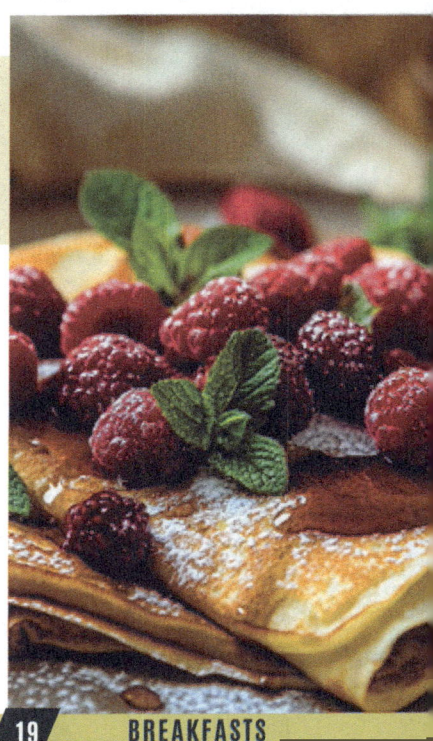

BREAKFASTS

TORTILLA BAKED EGGS

Ingredients:

- 2 tsp. olive oil (for brushing the pan)
- 2 small corn tortillas
- 1 cup/30g baby spinach, roughly chopped
- 2 tbsps./8g green leaves of scallions, finely chopped
- 6 large eggs
- 6 cherry tomatoes, quartered
- ¼ tsp. paprika
- Salt and pepper to taste
- 2 tbsps./15g vegan cheese (optional, grated)

Instructions:

1. Preheat the oven to 350°F/180°C. Prepare ingredients by chopping spinach, slicing scallion greens, quartering cherry tomatoes, and grating cheese if using.
2. Brush a small oven-proof skillet or baking dish with olive oil. The dish should be slightly smaller than the tortilla to allow the edges to curl up and form a lip. Press the tortilla gently into the dish.
3. Spread the chopped spinach evenly over the tortilla.
4. Crack the eggs on top of the spinach. Sprinkle with scallion greens and cherry tomatoes. Season with paprika, salt, and pepper. Add grated vegan cheese if desired.
5. Bake in the oven for 15–20 minutes or until the egg whites are set and no longer jiggle.
6. Remove from the oven then carefully transfer to a plate. Slice into quarters and serve warm.

Per serving:
Calories: 402kcal | Fat: 24g | Carbs: 19g | Protein: 25g | Fiber: 3g | Sugar: 4g

Medium | 2 Servings | 5 min | 15 min

BANANA MUFFINS

Ingredients:

- ½ cup/120g green banana, mashed
- ½ cup/65g gluten-free flour
- ¼ tsp. baking soda
- ¼ tsp. cinnamon
- 1 large egg
- 2 tbsp. olive oil
- 1 tbsp./15ml pure maple syrup

Instructions:

1. Preheat the oven to 350°F/180°C. Line a 4-cup muffin tin with paper liners.
2. In your bowl, mix mashed green banana, egg, olive oil, and maple syrup.
3. In another bowl, combine gluten-free flour, baking soda, and cinnamon. Drizzle the dry ingredients to the wet mixture and stir until smooth.
4. Spoon batter into muffin cups, filling each halfway.
5. Bake for 18–20 minutes or until a toothpick inserted into the center comes out clean. Cool before serving.

Per serving:
Calories: 260kcal | Fat: 8g | Carbs: 31g | Protein: 4g | Fiber: 3g | Sugar: 8g

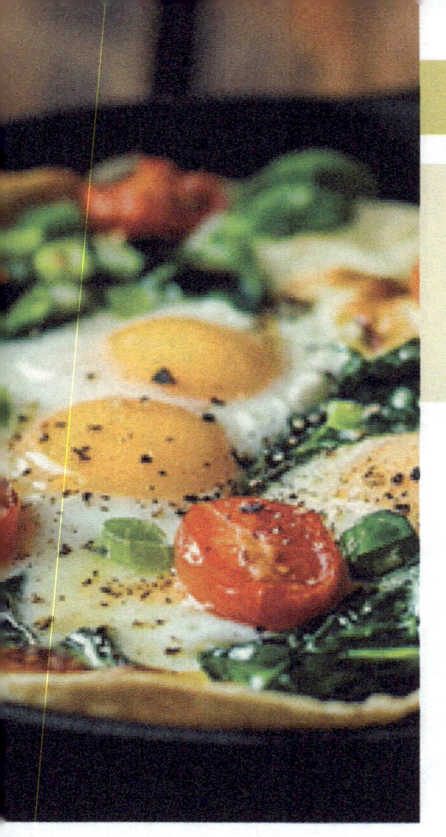

Medium | 2 Servings | 10 min | 20 min

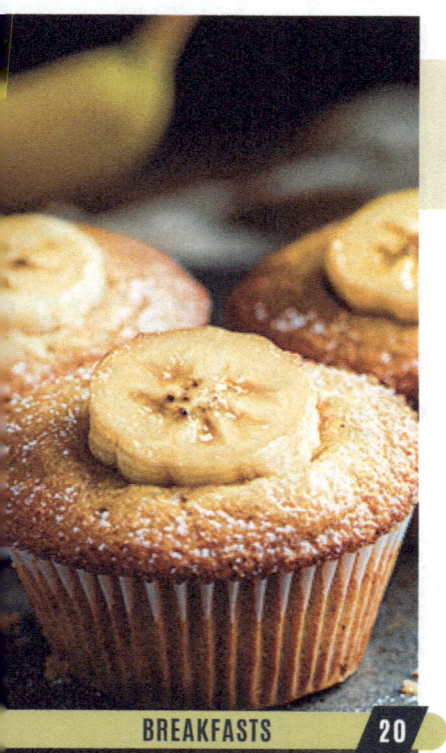

BREAKFASTS

TROPICAL MILLET PORRIDGE

Ingredients:

- ⅔ cup/100g hulled millet seed
- 1 ⅔ cups/400ml boiling water
- Pinch of salt
- ⅔ cup/160ml lactose-free milk or almond milk
- 2 tbsps./20g dried shredded coconut
- ⅓ cup/50g strawberries (2-3 medium strawberries)
- ½ banana
- Pinch of cinnamon
- 2 tsps./10ml apple syrup

Instructions:

1. Toast the millet seed in a saucepan over medium-high heat for about 2-3 minutes, or until it turns golden.
2. Add boiling water and a pinch of salt.
3. Cover and reduce heat to low, simmering for 15-20 minutes until most of the water is absorbed and the millet is soft.
4. Let the porridge to stand for 5 minutes.
5. Peel and slice the banana, then cut the strawberries into quarters.
6. Once the millet is cooked, stir in your choice of lactose-free milk until creamy. Add more milk if needed. Mix in the shredded coconut and a pinch of cinnamon.
7. Divide the porridge between two bowls. Top with sliced banana, strawberries, and a drizzle of maple syrup.

Per serving:
Calories: 515kcal | Fat: 18g | Carbs: 57g | Protein: 12g | Fiber: 10g | Sugar: 10g

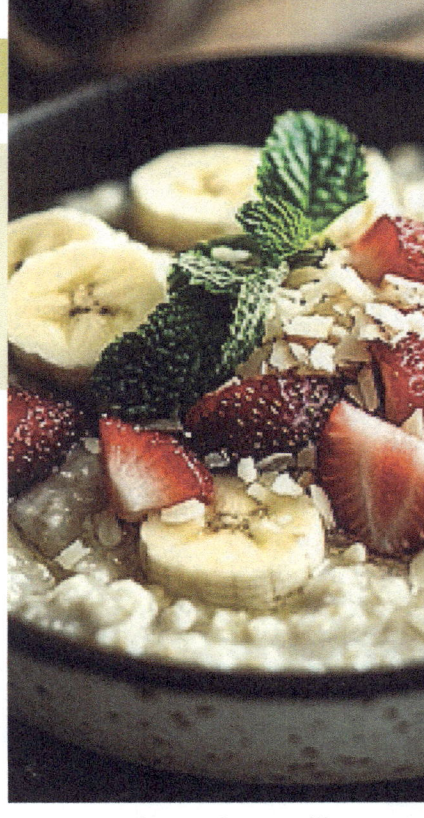

Medium | 2 Servings | 5 min | 30 min

GRILLED ZUCCHINI WITH POACHED EGGS

Medium | 2 Servings | 5 min | 10 min

Ingredients:

- 2 medium zucchinis, sliced into rounds
- 2 large eggs
- 1 tbsp. olive oil
- Salt and pepper to taste
- Fresh herbs (optional for garnish, such as parsley)

Instructions:

1. Preheat the grill pan to medium heat.
2. Toss zucchini rounds with salt, olive oil, and pepper. Grill for 3–4 minutes per side, until tender and lightly charred.
3. Meanwhile, poach the eggs by bringing water to a simmer in a saucepan. Add eggs gently and cook for 3–4 minutes, until the whites are set.
4. Plate the grilled zucchini and top with poached eggs. Garnish using fresh herbs if desired and serve warm.

Per serving:
Calories: 260kcal | Fat: 14g | Carbs: 7g | Protein: 13g | Fiber: 3g | Sugar: 4g

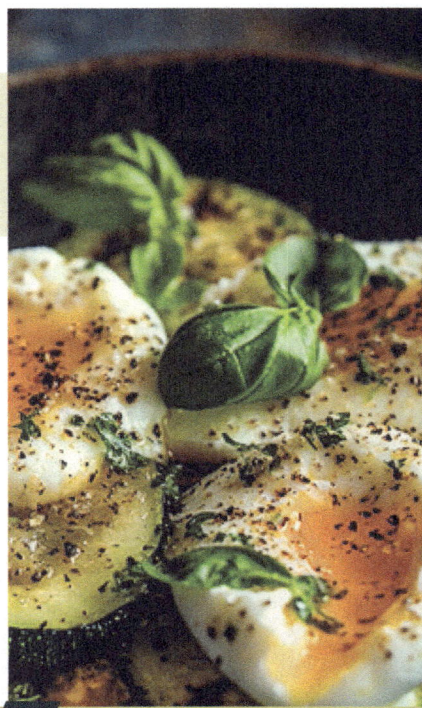

BREAKFASTS

MAPLE GRANOLA

Ingredients:

- 1 tbsp./8–10g almonds, roughly chopped
- 2 tbsps./12g rolled oats
- 2 tsps./6g buckwheat kernels
- 1 tsp. linseeds/flaxseeds
- 1 tsp. sunflower seeds
- 1 tsp. pepitas (pumpkin seeds)
- 1 tsp. chia seeds
- 1/8 tsp. ground cinnamon
- 1 tsp./5ml maple syrup
- 1 tsp. coconut oil
- 1 tsp. extra virgin olive oil
- 1 tsp. natural peanut butter
- 1/8 tsp./0.5ml vanilla essence

Instructions:

1. Preheat your oven to 320°F/160°C fan-forced (or 356°F/180°C for a conventional oven). Line a baking tray with baking paper.
2. In your bowl, mix all dry ingredients: almonds, oats, buckwheat, linseeds, sunflower seeds, chia seeds, pepitas, and cinnamon.
3. In a microwave-safe jug, combine maple syrup, coconut oil, olive oil, peanut butter, and vanilla essence. Heat until fully melted.
4. Place the wet mixture over the dry ingredients and stir until evenly coated. Spread the granola mixture thinly on the prepared tray, pressing it down firmly to help it stick and get crunchy.
5. Bake for 12–18 minutes, or until lightly golden. Remove from the oven and let cool completely.
6. Once cooled, break into clusters and store in an airtight container for up to 4 weeks.

Per serving:
Calories: 228kcal | Fat: 12g | Carbs: 12g | Protein: 5g | Fiber: 3g | Sugar: 6g

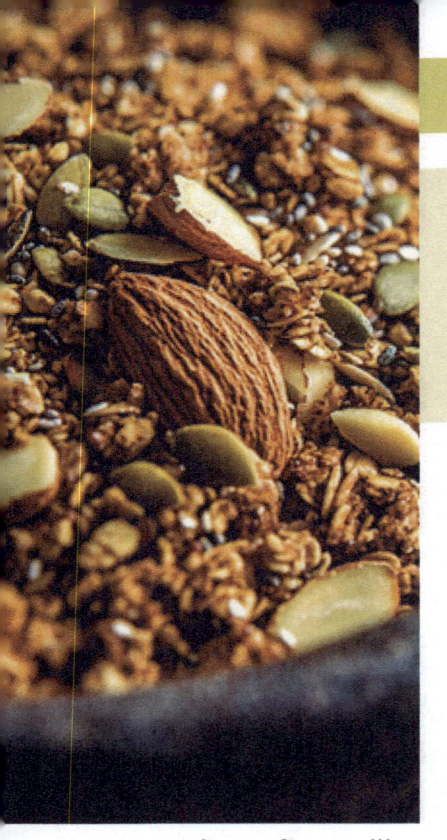

Medium | 2 Servings | 5 min | 18 min

PUMPKIN COCONUT MILK SMOOTHIE

Easy | 2 Servings | 5 min | None

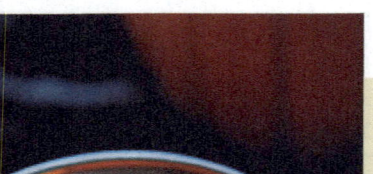

Ingredients:

- ½ cup/120g pumpkin puree
- ½ cup/120ml coconut milk (unsweetened)
- ½ tsp. cinnamon
- 1 tbsp./15ml maple syrup (optional for sweetness)
- Ice cubes (optional)

Instructions:

1. Combine pumpkin puree, coconut milk, cinnamon, and maple syrup (if using) in a blender.
2. Blend until smooth.
3. Include ice cubes if desired for a chilled smoothie, then blend again until the desired consistency is reached.
4. Serve immediately in chilled glasses.

Per serving:
Calories: 230kcal | Fat: 12g | Carbs: 22g | Protein: 2g | Fiber: 5g | Sugar: 7g

BREAKFASTS

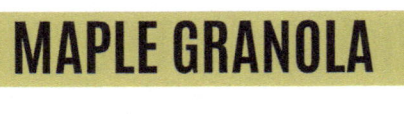

Chapter 3:
THE THREE S'S:
Salads, Soups, and Sides

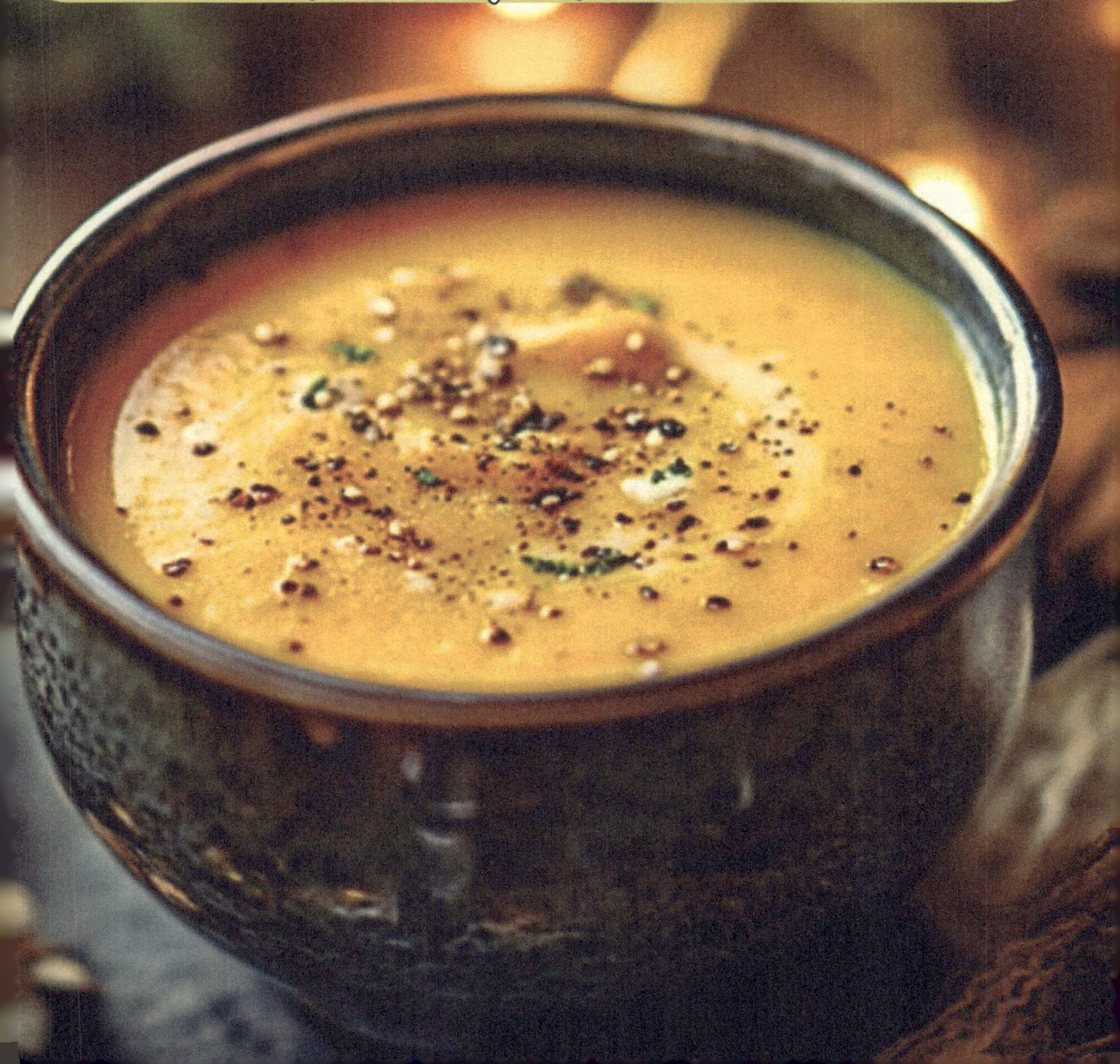

GRAPEFRUIT PRAWN SALAD

Medium | 2 Servings | 10 min | 10 min

Ingredients:

- 1 ½ cups/200g peeled, cooked prawns (about 8-10 prawns)
- ½ pink grapefruit, peeled and segmented
- ¼ long green chili, sliced
- ¼ cup/10g fresh mint leaves
- 1 Lebanese cucumber, cut thinly on the diagonal (about 1 ½ cups/180g)
- ⅛ cup/5g coriander leaves
- ¼ cup/20g shredded coconut
- ¼ cup/35g roasted peanuts
- 1 tsp. caster sugar
- ¼ cup/60ml lime juice (about 1 lime)
- 1 tbsp./15ml fish sauce

Instructions:

1. Heat a small pan set to medium heat. Add the prawns and cook for about 2-3 minutes until they turn pink and opaque. Remove from heat and let them cool slightly.
2. In a large bowl, combine the prawns, grapefruit, chili, mint, coriander, cucumber, shredded coconut, and peanuts.
3. To make the dressing, whisk together the sugar, lime juice, and fish sauce.
4. Drizzle the dressing over the salad then gently toss to mix everything together.
5. Serve immediately, arranging the salad mixture on a plate.

Per serving:
Calories: 367 kcal | Fat: 16g | Carbs: 10g | Protein: 27g | Fiber: 7g | Sugar: 9g

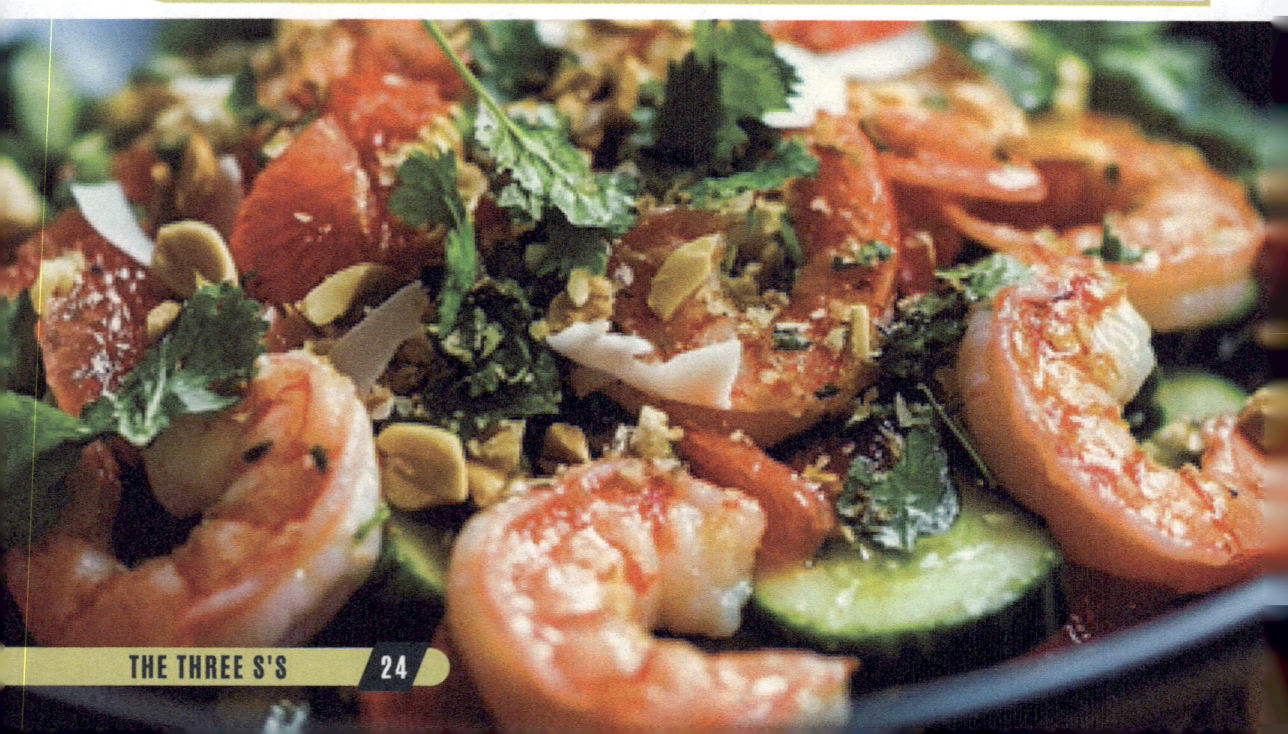

MAPLE GLAZED BABY CARROTS

Ingredients:

- 1 ½ tbsps./21g salted butter
- 8 medium-sized baby carrots, trimmed and scrubbed
- 2 ½ tbsps./38ml pure maple syrup
- ¼ cup/60ml freshly squeezed orange juice
- ½ tsp./2g orange zest
- ¼ tsp. salt
- ¼ tsp. cracked black pepper
- ½ tbsp. mustard
- ½ tbsp. chopped herbs of your choice (thyme, parsley, chives, basil)

Instructions:

1. In a large non-stick sauté pan, melt the butter over high heat.
2. Add the carrots, maple syrup, orange juice, orange zest, mustard (if using), salt, and pepper. Gently mix to coat the carrots, then bring the mixture to a boil.
3. Cover the pan using a tight-fitting lid, reduce the heat, then simmer for about 4 minutes.
4. Remove the lid and stir occasionally for about 15 minutes until the carrots are tender, adding more water if needed if the liquid reduces too much.
5. Once tender, remove from heat and garnish with your choice of herbs. Serve immediately.

Per serving:
Calories: 290kcal | Fat: 12g | Carbs: 24g | Protein: 5g | Fiber: 7g | Sugar: 14g

Easy | 2 Servings | 5 min | 20 min

CAPRESE SALAD

Easy | 2 Servings | 5 min | None

Ingredients:

- 1 ¼ cups/185g cherry tomatoes
- 4 cherry bocconcini, sliced
- 2 tbsps. torn basil leaves
- Salt & pepper, to taste
- 1 tbsp. extra virgin olive oil, to serve
- 1 tbsp./15ml balsamic vinegar, to serve

Instructions:

1. Cut the cherry tomatoes in halves or slices. Place them in a serving bowl.
2. Add the sliced bocconcini and torn basil leaves on top of the tomatoes. Sprinkle using salt and pepper to taste, then gently toss together.
3. Just before serving, drizzle the olive oil and balsamic vinegar over the salad.

Per serving:
Calories: 183 kcal | Fat: 10g | Carbs: 2g | Protein: 6g | Fiber: 1g | Sugar: 1g

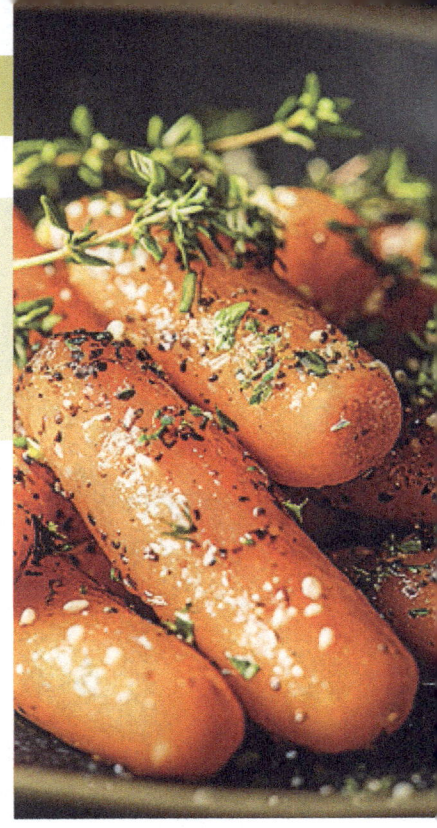

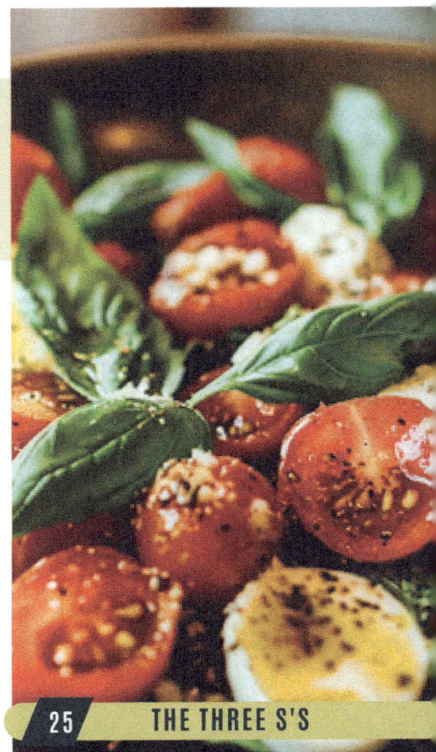

ZUCCHINI AND BELL PEPPER SALAD

Ingredients:

- 2 medium zucchinis, sliced into rounds
- 1 green bell pepper, sliced
- 1 tbsp. olive oil
- 1 tbsp./15ml fresh lemon juice
- Salt and pepper to taste
- 1 tbsp. fresh basil, chopped

Instructions:

1. Preheat the grill pan set to medium heat.
2. Toss the zucchini and bell pepper slices with olive oil, salt, and pepper.
3. Grill the vegetables for 3–4 minutes per side until tender and lightly charred.
4. Once grilled, transfer to a serving plate, drizzle using fresh lemon juice, and sprinkle with fresh basil.
5. Serve warm or at room temperature.

Easy | 2 Servings | 10 min | 10 min

Per serving:
Calories: 200kcal | Fat: 10g | Carbs: 14g | Protein: 3g | Fiber: 5g | Sugar: 7g

SPINACH-ORANGE SALAD WITH NUTS

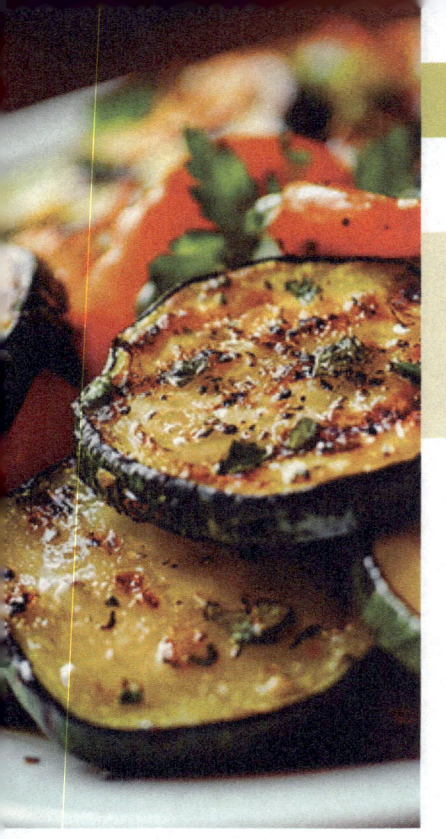

Easy | 2 Servings | 5 min | None

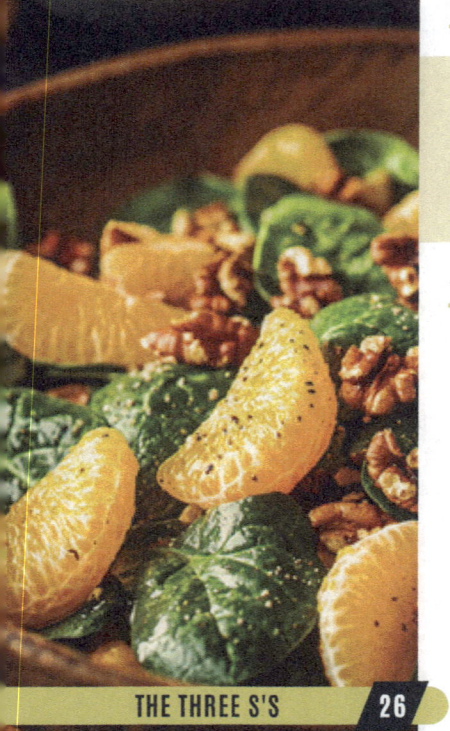

Ingredients:

- 4 cups/120g fresh spinach leaves
- 1 orange, peeled and sliced
- ¼ cup/30g walnuts, toasted
- 1 tbsp. olive oil
- 1 tbsp./15ml balsamic vinegar
- Salt and pepper to taste

Instructions:

1. In a large bowl, toss together the fresh spinach and orange slices.
2. Drizzle with olive oil and balsamic vinegar.
3. Sprinkle with toasted walnuts and season with salt and pepper.
4. Serve immediately as a refreshing, light salad.

Per serving:
Calories: 210kcal | Fat: 14g | Carbs: 14g | Protein: 3g | Fiber: 4g | Sugar: 8g

THE THREE S'S

PARMESAN AND THYME PARSNIPS

Ingredients:

- 3 tbsps./45g polenta (cornmeal)
- ½ cup/50g grated Parmesan
- 1 ½ tsps. thyme leaves
- 2 ½ cups/300g parsnips, quartered and cored
- 3 tbsps. olive oil
- 1 ½ tbsps. chopped parsley

Instructions:

1. Preheat the oven to 425°F/220°C.
2. In a large bowl, combine the polenta, Parmesan, and thyme, then set aside.
3. Bring a pot of salted water to a boil, add the parsnips, and cook for 6 minutes or until just tender. Drain well.
4. While the parsnips are still hot, toss them in the Parmesan mixture, ensuring they are evenly coated. In a roasting pan, heat the olive oil over the stove.
5. Add the parsnips then toss them to coat in the oil.
6. Transfer the roasting pan to the oven then roast the parsnips for 30 minutes, turning them halfway through for even cooking.
7. Once done, sprinkle with chopped parsley and serve immediately.

Per serving:
Calories: 390 kcal | Fat: 18g | Carbs: 28g | Protein: 9g | Fiber: 8g | Sugar: 10g

Medium 2 Servings 20 min 40 min

VEGETABLE & CHICKPEA SOUP

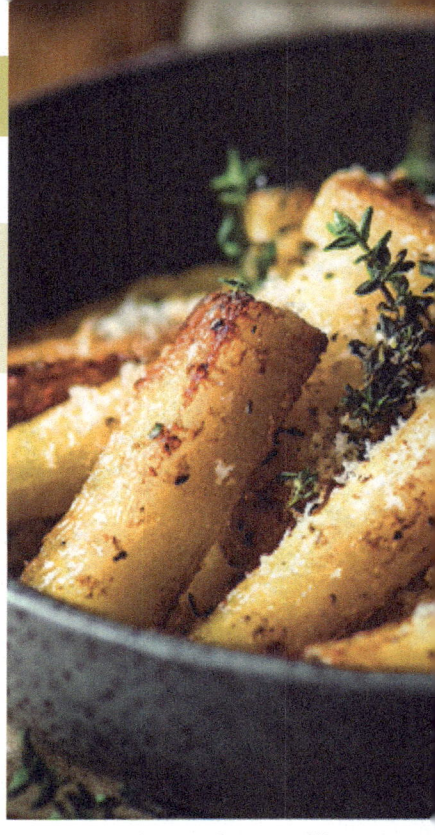

Medium 2 Servings 10 min 30 min

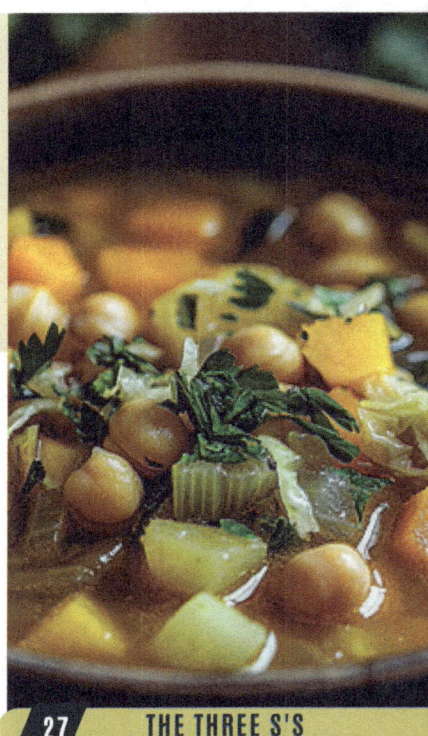

Ingredients:

- 2 tbsps. garlic-infused oil (see recipe p.70)
- 1 cup/90g green leek leaves (diced, green parts only)
- 4 cups/960ml water (add more if needed)
- ½ cup/85g canned chickpeas, drained and rinsed well
- 1 medium carrot, diced
- 1 medium potato, diced
- 1 cup/200g pumpkin, diced
- ½ cup/45g shredded cabbage
- ½ cup/60g green beans, chopped
- 2 tbsps. fresh parsley, chopped
- Salt and black pepper, to taste

Instructions:

1. Heat the garlic-infused oil in a large pot over medium heat. Sauté the leek leaves for 2-3 minutes until softened. Add the water and bring to a boil.
2. Stir in the carrot, potato, and pumpkin. Reduce heat to a simmer and cook for 15 minutes, or until the vegetables start to soften.
3. Add the cabbage, green beans, and chickpeas. Simmer for another 10 minutes, or until all the vegetables are tender. Stir in parsley, and season with salt and black pepper to taste. Serve warm.

Per serving:
Calories: 200kcal | Fat: 5g | Carbs: 30g | Protein: 5g | Fiber: 6g | Sugar: 12g

THE THREE S'S

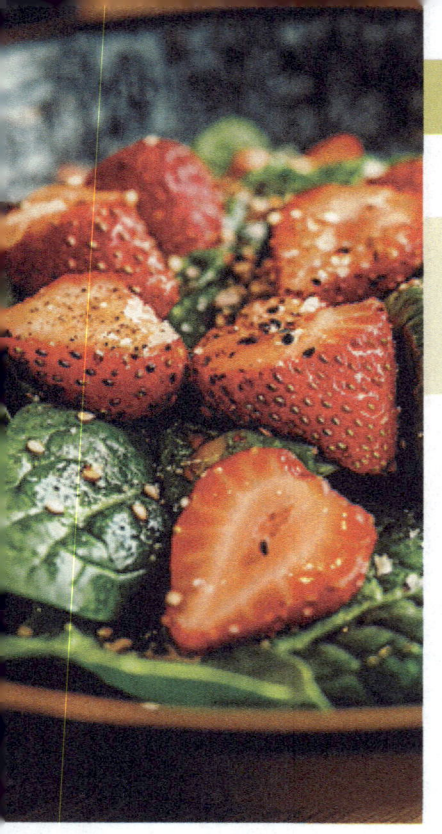

SPINACH SALAD WITH STRAWBERRIES

Ingredients:

- 4 cups/120g fresh baby spinach
- ½ cup/75g strawberries, sliced
- 1 tbsp. olive oil
- 1 tbsp./15ml balsamic vinegar
- Salt and pepper to taste

Instructions:

1. In your bowl, combine the baby spinach and sliced strawberries
2. Drizzle with olive oil and balsamic vinegar.
3. Toss gently to coat the spinach and strawberries in the dressing.
4. Season using salt and pepper, then serve immediately.

Easy | 2 Servings | 5 min | None

Per serving:
Calories: 150kcal | Fat: 8g | Carbs: 10g | Protein: 2g | Fiber: 3g | Sugar: 5g

Easy | 2 Servings | 5 min | None

BEANS AND CARROTS IN VINAIGRETTE

Ingredients:

- 1 cup/125g green beans, trimmed
- 1 cup/120g carrots, sliced
- 2 tbsps./30ml Lemon Vinaigrette (see recipe p.69)

Instructions:

1. Bring a saucepan of water to a boil. Add the green beans and carrots, cooking for about 5–7 minutes until tender.
2. Drain and rinse the vegetables under cold water to stop the cooking process.
3. Toss the cooked vegetables with the lemon vinaigrette.
4. Serve immediately or chill for later use.

Per serving:
Calories: 190 kcal | Fat: 10g | Carbs: 16g | Protein: 2g | Fiber: 5g | Sugar: 7g

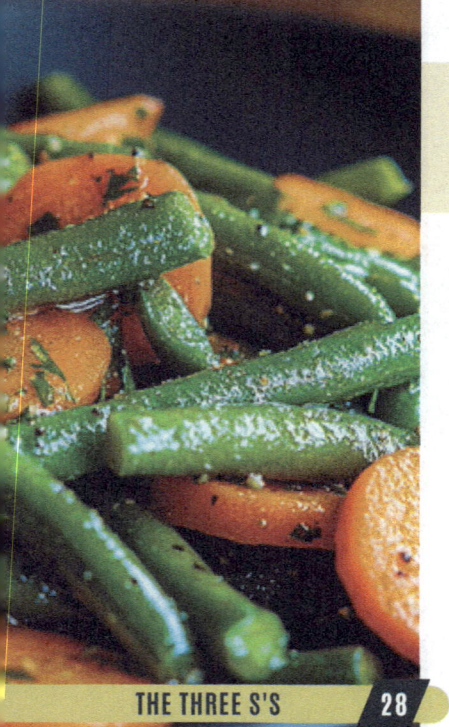

THE THREE S'S

CHICKEN RAMEN NOODLE SOUP

Medium | **2 Servings** | **15 min** | **45 min**

Ingredients:

- 2 small chicken breast fillets (about 200g)
- 2 tsps. garlic-infused olive oil
- 2 tsps. sesame oil
- 2 tsps. fresh ginger, minced
- 2 tbsps./30ml tamari soy sauce
- 1 ½ tbsps./22.5ml rice wine vinegar
- 2 tsps. white sugar
- 2 large eggs
- 4 cups/960ml low-FODMAP chicken stock
- 1 bunch bok choy, separated into pieces (about 200g)
- ½ cup/75g green spring onion tops, finely chopped
- 3 ½ oz./100g dry rice noodles or soba noodles
- Salt and pepper, to taste

Instructions:

1. Preheat oven to 375°F/190°C.
2. Season chicken breasts with salt and pepper. Heat olive oil and garlic in a large oven-safe skillet over medium heat. Add chicken breasts and cook for 5 minutes on each side until golden. Transfer skillet to oven and bake for 15-20 minutes, or until cooked through. Remove chicken from skillet, cover with foil and set aside.
3. While chicken is baking, heat sesame oil in a large saucepan over medium heat. Add minced ginger and cook for 2-3 minutes until softened. Add soy sauce, rice wine vinegar and sugar and cook for another minute. Add low FODMAP chicken broth, cover and bring to a simmer. Once boiling, remove the lid and let it simmer for 5 minutes. Add the bok choy and cook for another 3-4 minutes until wilted. Season with salt to taste.
4. In a separate saucepan, bring the water to a boil. Carefully add the eggs and simmer for 8 minutes until soft-boiled. Then transfer them to cold water. Once cool, peel and cut in half lengthwise. Slice the fried chicken into thin slices. In a saucepan, bring the water to a boil and add the noodles. Cook the noodles for 2-3 minutes, or until tender.
5. Divide the noodles between two bowls, then top with the shredded chicken, ramen broth, green onion tops, and soft-boiled eggs. Serve immediately.

Per serving:
Calories: 630 kcal | Fat: 18g | Carbs: 46g | Protein: 54g | Fiber: 2g | Sugar: 8g

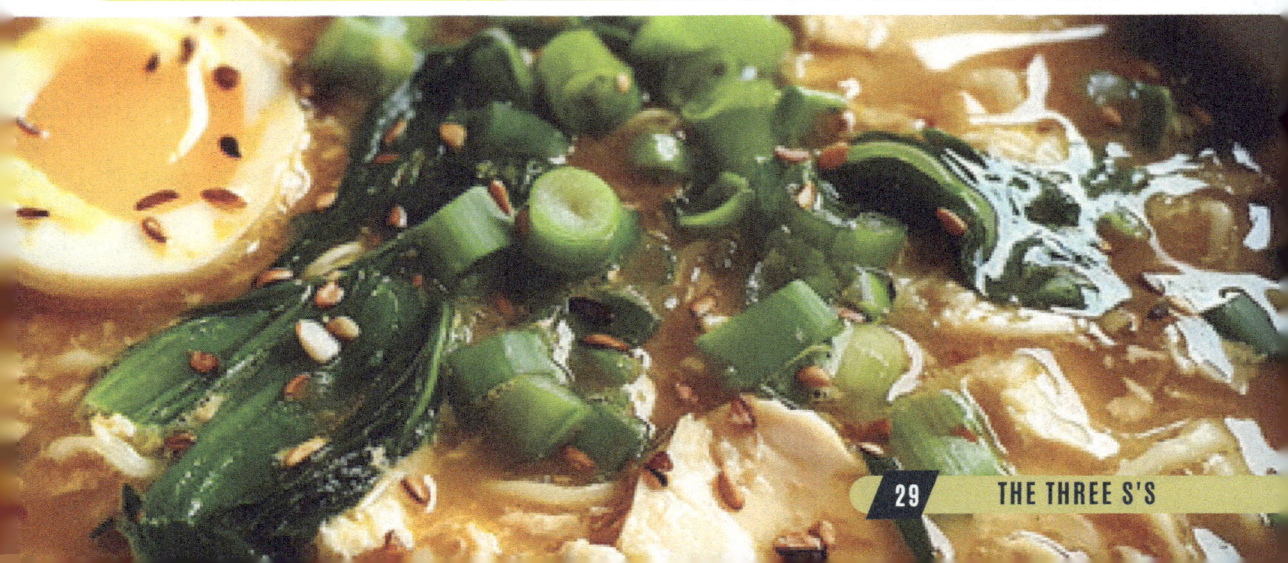

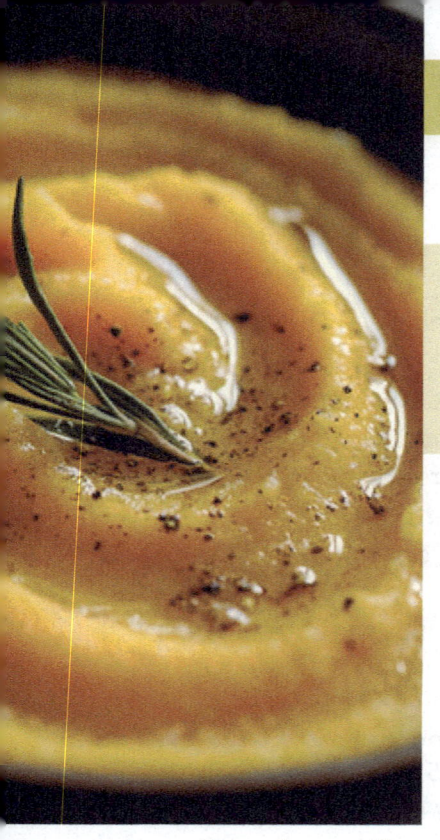

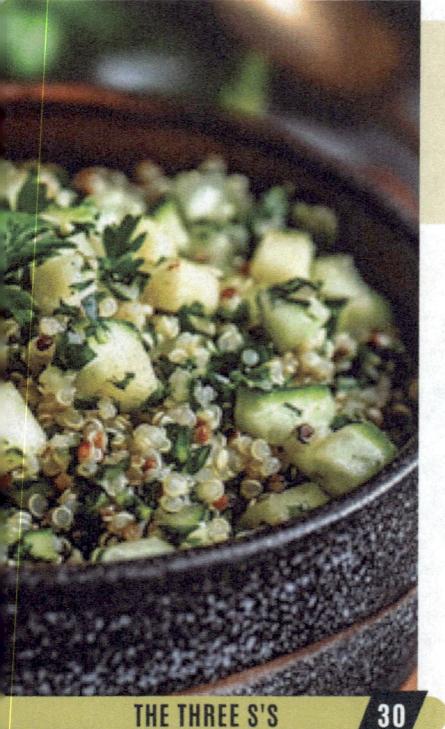

CARROT AND PARSNIP PUREE

Ingredients:

- 2 medium carrots, peeled and chopped
- 2 medium parsnips, peeled and chopped
- 1 tbsp. olive oil
- Salt and pepper to taste
- ¼ cup/60ml lactose-free milk (optional for creaminess)

Instructions:

1. In a saucepan, boil a pot of water. Add the chopped carrots and parsnips, cooking for 15-20 minutes until tender.
2. Drain the vegetables and transfer to a blender or use a hand masher to mash until smooth.
3. Add olive oil, salt, and pepper. For extra creaminess, add lactose-free milk.
4. Blend or mash until you reach your desired texture and serve warm.

Per serving:
Calories: 200 kcal | Fat: 8g | Carbs: 20g | Protein: 2g | Fiber: 5g | Sugar: 8g

Easy | 2 Servings | 10 min | 20 min

Easy | 2 Servings | 10 min | 15 min

QUINOA TABBOULEH WITH CUCUMBER

Ingredients:

- ½ cup/90g quinoa (rinsed)
- 1 cup/240ml water
- ½ cucumber, diced
- 1 tbsp. olive oil
- Salt and pepper to taste
- ½ cup/15g fresh parsley, chopped
- 1 tbsp./15ml fresh lemon juice

Instructions:

1. In a saucepan, boil a 1 cup of water. Stir in the quinoa, then lower the heat to a simmer. Cover and cook for 12–15 minutes, until the water is absorbed, and the quinoa is tender.
2. Remove the pan from the heat then fluff the quinoa with a fork. Allow it to cool to room temperature.
3. In a large bowl, combine the cooled quinoa, cucumber, and parsley.
4. Drizzle using olive oil and lemon juice, then season with salt and pepper to taste.
5. Toss to combine and serve.

Per serving:
Calories: 250kcal | Fat: 8g | Carbs: 28g | Protein: 6g | Fiber: 4g | Sugar: 3g

THE THREE S'S

SALTBUSH DUKKAH

Ingredients:

- 2 tbsps. dried ground saltbush leaves
- ⅓ cup/50g finely chopped macadamias
- 2 tbsps. sesame seeds
- 2 tbsps. roughly chopped pumpkin seeds/pepitas
- 2 tsps. coriander seeds
- 1 tsp. cumin seeds
- ⅓ tsp. ground peppercorns

Instructions:

1. In a fry pan, toast the macadamias, sesame seeds, and pumpkin seeds set to medium heat for about 2 minutes, continuously stirring to prevent burning. Once toasted, remove from heat and let cool in a bowl.
2. Place the saltbush leaves, cumin seeds, coriander seeds, and peppercorns into the fry pan. Toast for 1-2 minutes, or until browned, and then remove from heat to cool.
3. Once the toasted ingredients have cooled, combine them in a bowl, stirring until well mixed.
4. Serve with salads, soups, dips, or as a crust for meats or fish.

Per serving:
Calories: 312 kcal | Fat: 24g | Carbs: 2g | Protein: 5g | Fiber: 4g | Sugar: 1g

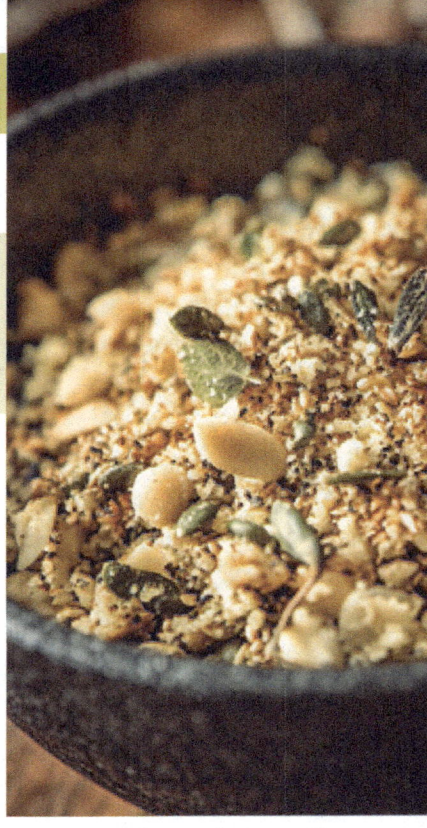

Medium | 2 Servings | 5 min | 15 min

SWEET POTATO WITH ROSEMARY

Medium | 2 Servings | 10 min | 30 min

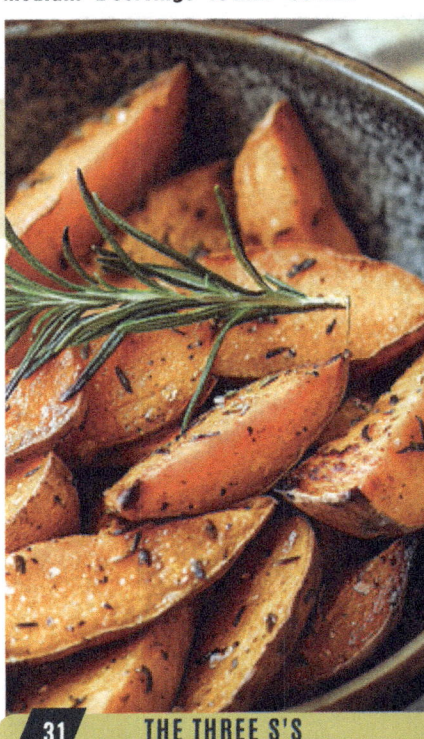

Ingredients:

- 2 medium sweet potatoes, peeled and cut into wedges (approximately 500g)
- 1 tbsp. olive oil
- 1 tbsp. fresh rosemary, chopped
- Salt and pepper to taste

Instructions:

1. Preheat the oven to 425°F/220°C.
2. In a bowl, toss the sweet potato wedges with olive oil, fresh rosemary, salt, and pepper until evenly coated.
3. Arrange the wedges in a single layer on a baking sheet.
4. Roast in the oven for 25–30 minutes, flipping halfway through, until the edges are golden brown and crispy.
5. Serve warm as a flavorful side dish, paired with Garlic-Infused Mayo Dipping Sauce (see recipe p.69).

Per serving:
Calories: 250 kcal | Fat: 9g | Carbs: 32g | Protein: 3g | Fiber: 5g | Sugar: 7g

NICOISE SALAD WITH TUNA

Ingredients:

- 1 ¼ cups/150g green beans, halved lengthways
- 1 boiled potato, chopped (about 1 ½ cups/225g)
- 1 ½ cups/45g butter lettuce, shredded
- 2 tbsps./20g black/green pitted olives, halved
- 6 cherry tomatoes, halved
- 2 anchovy fillets (marinated in oil and salt only), drained and chopped
- 1 can (170g) tuna in oil
- 1 tsp. mustard
- 2 tsps./10ml rice wine vinegar
- 2 hard-boiled eggs, halved

Instructions:

1. Place the diced potato in a saucepan with cold water. Bring to a boil, then reduce heat to low and cover. Simmer for 12-15 minutes until the potato is fork-tender. Drain and set aside.
2. Place the green beans to a bowl and pour boiling water over them. Let them sit for 1 minute, or until they turn bright green and are slightly tender. Drain, rinse using cold water, and drain again. In a large bowl, combine the olives, lettuce, green beans, cherry tomatoes, anchovy, tuna (undrained), mustard, and rice wine vinegar. Add the boiled potato and gently toss to combine. Season with salt and pepper to taste.
3. Top the salad with halved hard-boiled eggs and serve immediately.

Per serving:
Calories: 600kcal | Fat: 28g | Carbs: 34g | Protein: 36g | Fiber: 8g | Sugar: 6g

Medium | 2 Servings | 5 min | 20 min

SPAGHETTI SQUASH WITH OLIVE OIL

Ingredients:

- 1 small spaghetti squash (approximately 700g)
- 1 tbsp. olive oil
- Salt and pepper to taste
- 1 tbsp. fresh basil, chopped

Instructions:

1. Preheat the oven to 400°F/200°C.
2. Cut the spaghetti squash in half lengthwise then scoop out the seeds.
3. Brush the cut sides of the squash with olive oil and sprinkle with salt and pepper.
4. Place the halves cut side down on a baking sheet then roast for 35–40 minutes, or until the squash is tender.
5. After roasting, use a fork to scrape out the strands, creating a spaghetti-like texture.
6. Transfer the strands to a bowl, toss with fresh basil, and serve warm.

Per serving:
Calories: 200kcal | Fat: 10g | Carbs: 16g | Protein: 3g | Fiber: 5g | Sugar: 4g

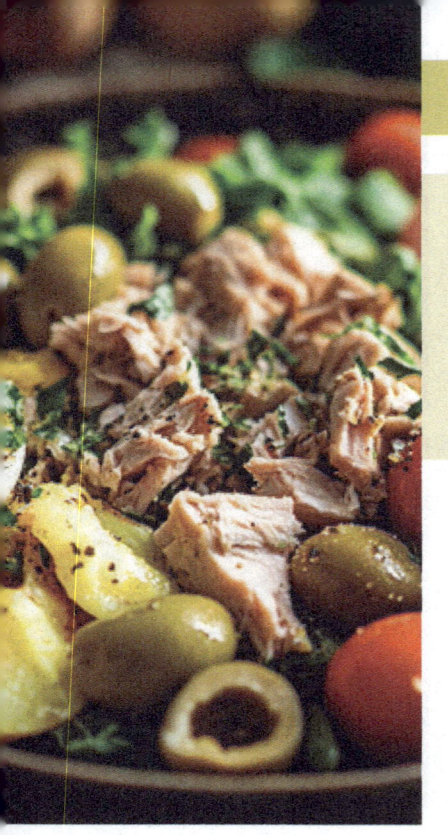

Medium | 2 Servings | 15 min | 40 min

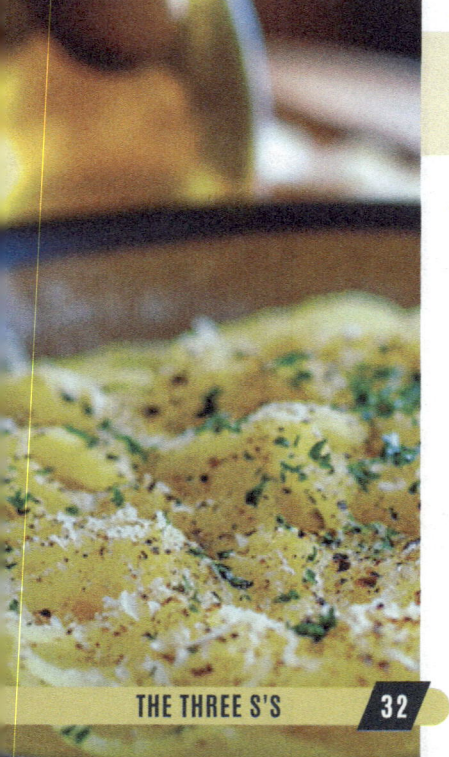

THE THREE S'S

Chapter 4: Flavor-Packed Main Dishes

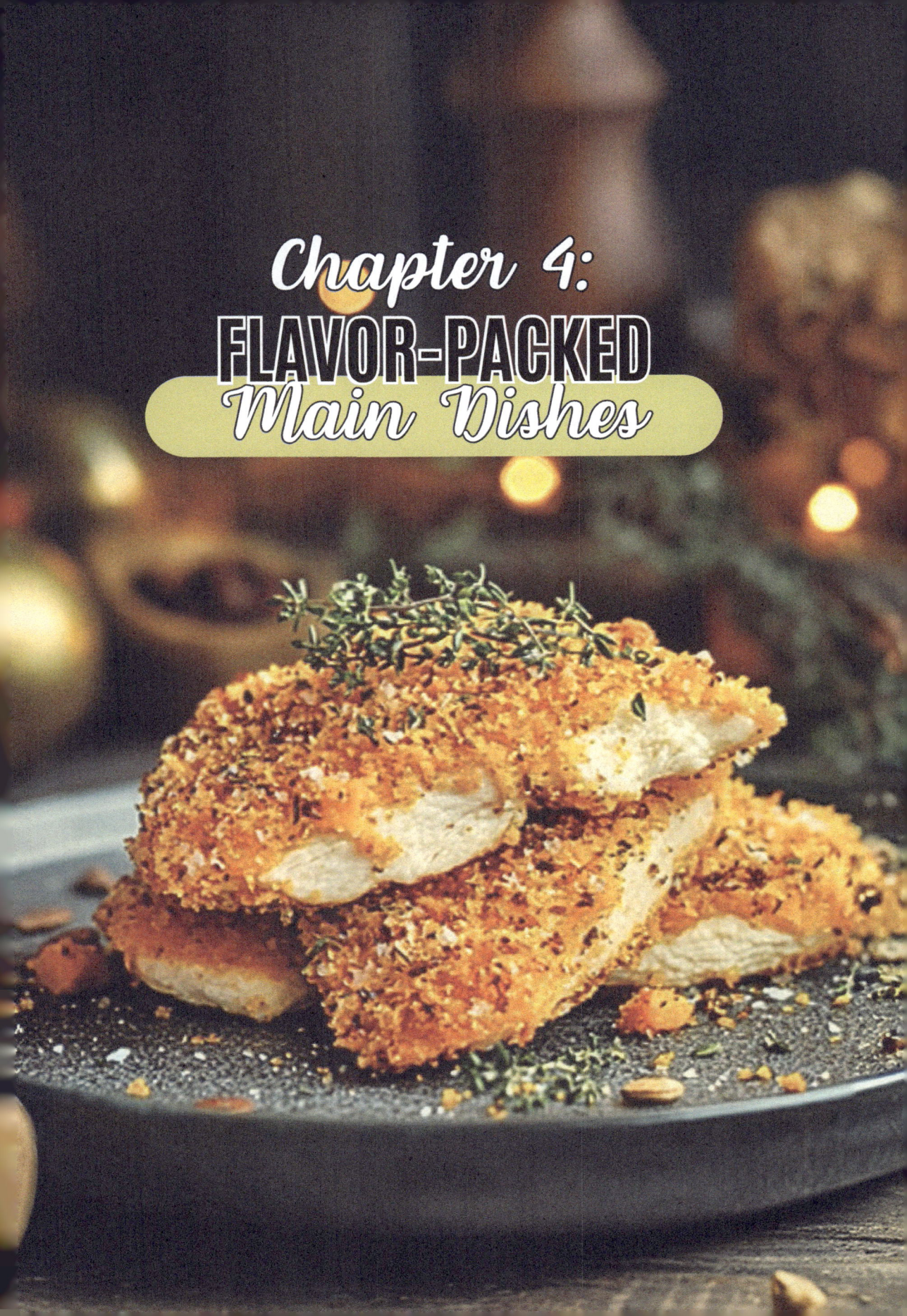

QUINOA-STUFFED BELL PEPPERS

Medium | 2 Servings | 15 min | 30 min

Ingredients:

- 2 large bell peppers, tops cut off and seeds removed
- ½ cup/90g quinoa
- 1 cup/240ml Homemade Chicken Stock (see recipe p.70)
- 1 tbsp. olive oil
- ½ cup/60g spinach, chopped
- ¼ cup/30g pumpkin seeds
- Salt and pepper to taste

Instructions:

1. Preheat the oven to 375°F/190°C.
2. Cook the quinoa using the package directions, using chicken stock for extra flavor.
3. While the quinoa is cooking, heat olive oil in a pan over medium heat. Place the spinach then cook for about 2 minutes, or until wilted.
4. Combine the cooked quinoa and spinach, then season with salt and pepper to taste. Stuff the mixture into the prepared bell peppers.
5. Bring the stuffed peppers in a baking dish and cover with foil.
6. Bake for 25-30 minutes, or until the peppers are tender.
7. Top with pumpkin seeds before serving and pair it with your favorite low-FODMAP side dishes.

Per serving:
Calories: 320kcal | Fat: 12g | Carbs: 32g | Protein: 9g | Fiber: 5g | Sugar: 5g

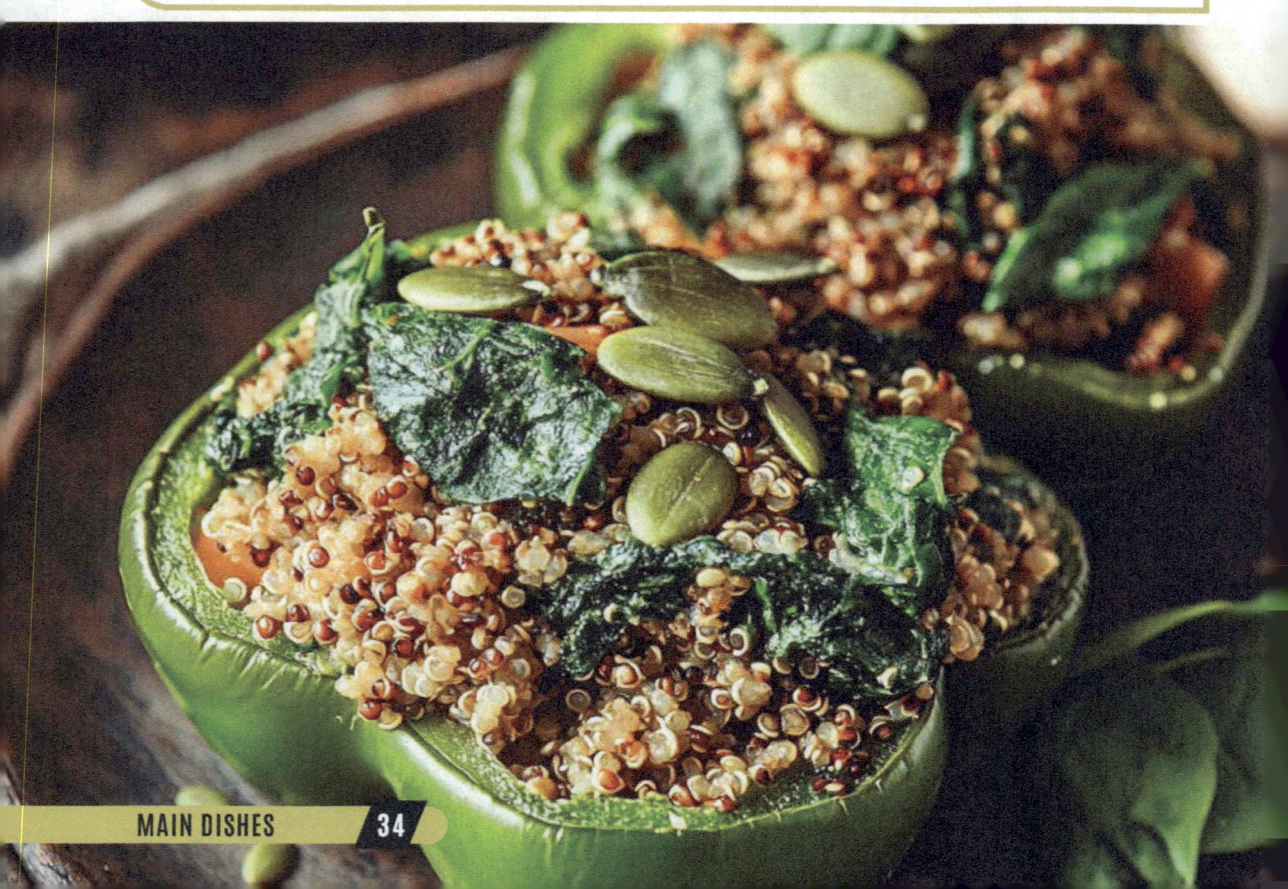

MAIN DISHES

GARLIC-INFUSED SHRIMP SKILLET

Ingredients:

- ½ lb./225g shrimp, peeled and deveined
- 1 tbsp. garlic-infused olive oil
- 1 tbsp./15ml fresh lemon juice
- Salt and pepper to taste
- Fresh parsley, chopped for garnish

Instructions:

1. Heat the garlic-infused olive oil in a skillet set to medium heat.
2. Add shrimp to the skillet then cook for 2-3 minutes on each side, or until the shrimp turns pink and opaque.
3. Season using salt, pepper, and fresh lemon juice.
4. Garnish using chopped parsley and serve immediately with a side of low-FODMAP vegetables or salad (refer to recipes in the previous chapter).

Per serving:
Calories: 270kcal | Fat: 14g | Carbs: 1g | Protein: 24g | Fiber: 1g | Sugar: 1g

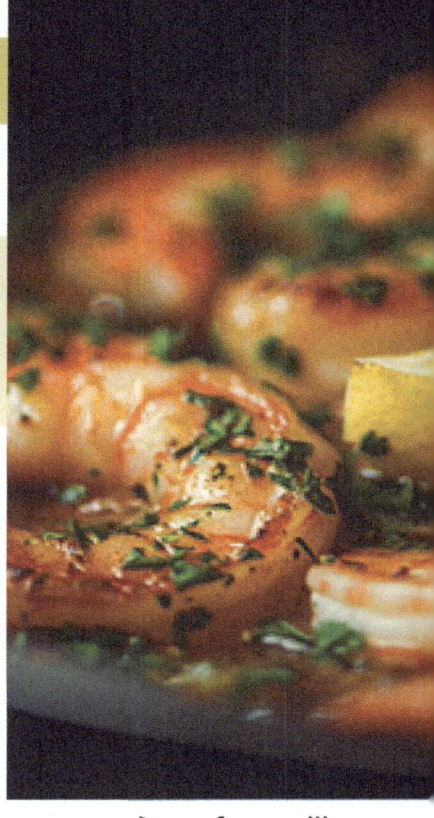

Easy | 2 Servings | 10 min | 5-7 min

OVEN-BAKED COD WITH LEMON

Easy | 2 Servings | 5 min | 15-20 min

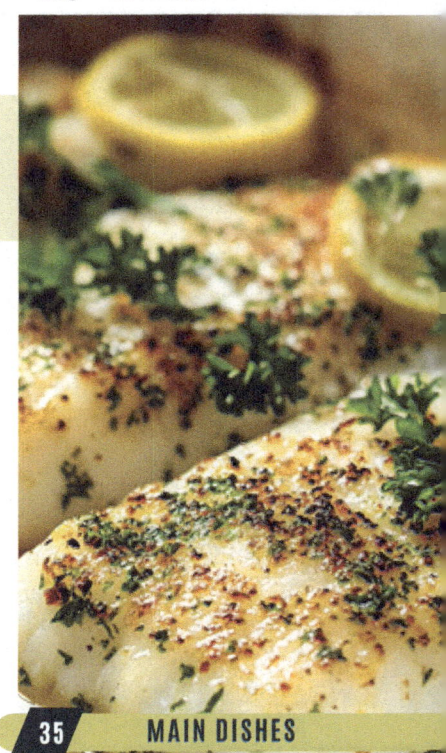

Ingredients:

- 2 cod fillets
- 1 tbsp. olive oil
- Juice of 1 lemon
- Fresh parsley, chopped
- Salt and pepper to taste

Instructions:

1. Preheat the oven to 375°F/190°C.
2. Arrange the cod fillets on a parchment-lined baking sheet.
3. Drizzle using olive oil and lemon juice, then season with salt and pepper.
4. Bake for 15-20 minutes, or until the fish easily flakes with a fork.
5. Top with fresh parsley and serve right away, paired with quinoa or with a side of low-FODMAP vegetables or salad (refer to recipes in the previous chapter).

Per serving:
Calories: 230 kcal | Fat: 8g | Carbs: 2g | Protein: 25g | Fiber: 0g | Sugar: 1g

MAIN DISHES

BEEF STIR-FRY WITH BROCCOLI

Ingredients:

- ½ lb./225g beef, thinly sliced (such as flank steak)
- 1 tbsp. Garlic-Infused Olive Oil (see recipe p.70)
- 1 tbsp. fresh ginger, grated
- ½ cup/50g broccoli florets
- ½ green bell pepper, thinly sliced
- 1 tbsp./15ml Ginger and Soy Marinade (see recipe p.69)
- Salt and pepper to taste

Instructions:

1. Heat the garlic-infused olive oil in a large skillet set to medium heat.
2. Add the sliced beef then cook for 3-4 minutes until browned.
3. Add the ginger, broccoli, and green bell pepper, and stir-fry for 3-4 minutes until vegetables are tender.
4. Stir in Ginger and Soy Marinade, salt, and pepper.
5. Serve immediately, garnished with sesame seeds or green onions if desired.
6. Pair with your favorite low-FODMAP side dishes.

Per serving:
Calories: 370 kcal | Fat: 18g | Carbs: 10g | Protein: 28g | Fiber: 4g | Sugar: 5g

Medium | 2 Servings | 10 min | 10 min

SWEET POTATO CRUSTED CHOPS

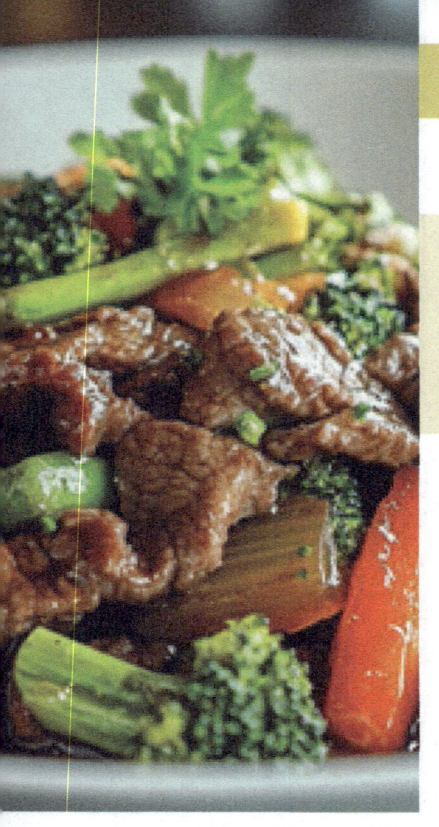

Medium | 2 Servings | 15 min | 20 min

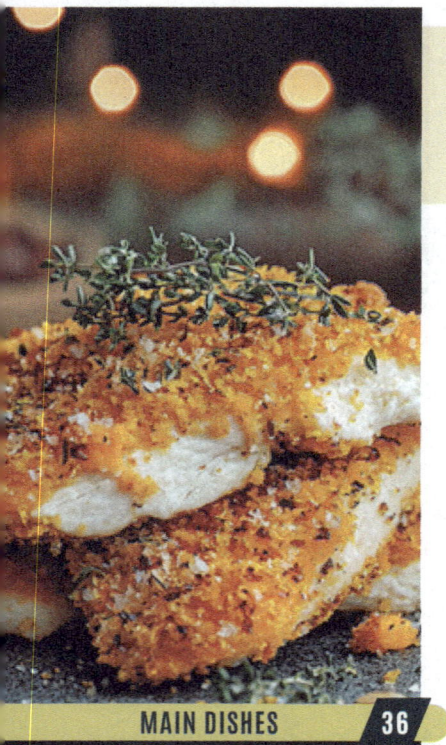

Ingredients:

- 2 chicken breast tenders
- 1 medium sweet potato, peeled and grated
- ½ cup/60g gluten-free breadcrumbs
- 1 tbsp. Garlic-Infused Olive Oil (see recipe p.70)
- 1 tsp. dried thyme
- Salt and pepper to taste

Instructions:

1. Preheat the oven to 400°F/200°C. Grate the sweet potato and squeeze out any excess moisture using a paper towel.
2. In a shallow bowl, mix grated sweet potato, breadcrumbs, thyme, salt, and pepper. Coat the chicken tenders in the mixture, pressing down to ensure an even crust.
3. Bring the chicken tenders on a baking sheet lined with parchment paper and drizzle with garlic-infused olive oil.
4. Bake for 18-20 minutes, flipping halfway through, until the chicken is cooked through then the crust is golden.
5. Serve with a side of roasted vegetables or with Garlic-Infused Mayo Dipping Sauce (see recipe p.69).

Per serving:
Calories: 320 kcal | Fat: 12g | Carbs: 20g | Protein: 28g | Fiber: 4g | Sugar: 4g

MAIN DISHES

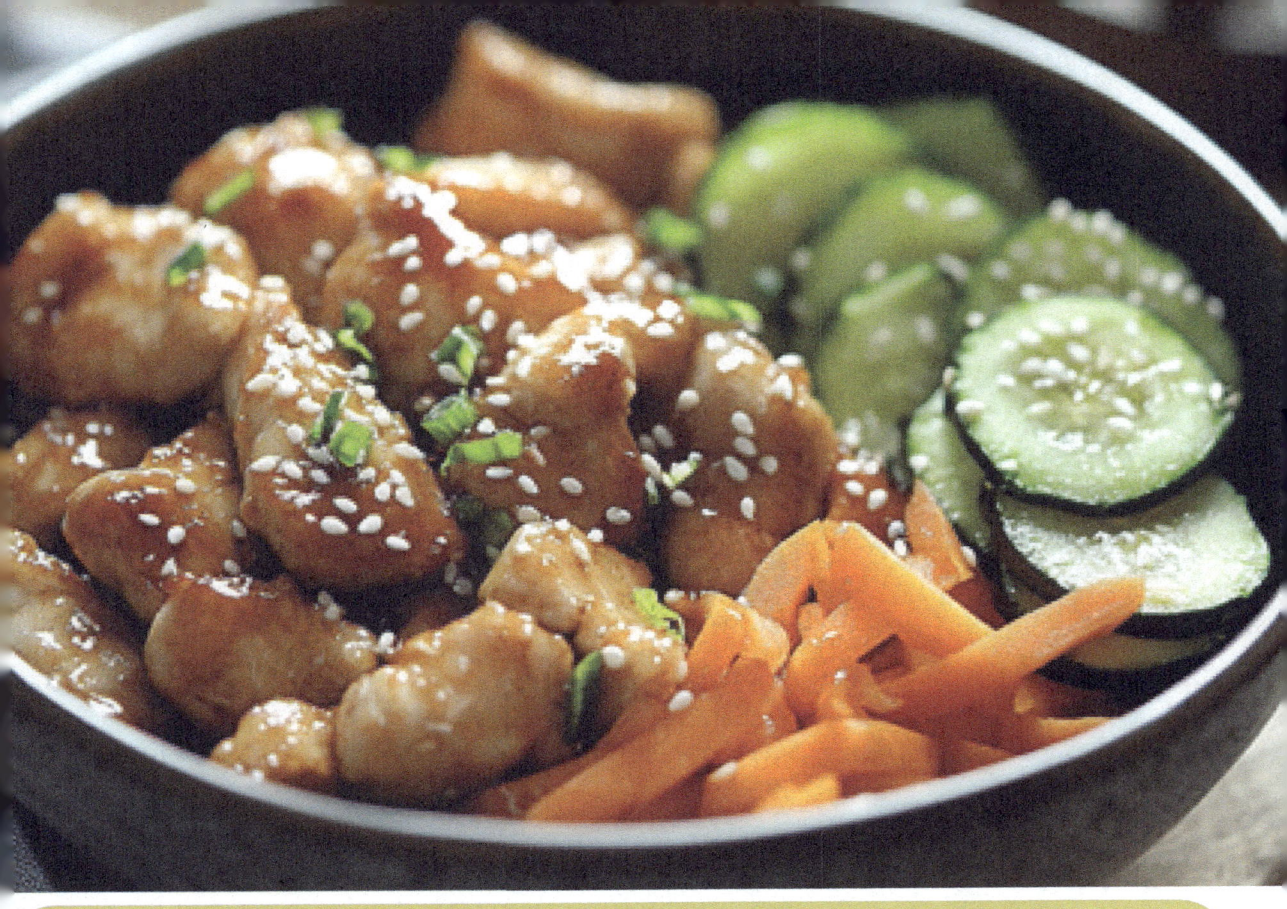

SESAME CHICKEN AND VEGETABLE BOWL

Medium | 2 Servings | 10 min | 10-12 min

Ingredients:

- 2 chicken breasts, thinly sliced
- 1 tbsp. Garlic-Infused Olive Oil (see recipe p.70)
- 1 tbsp. sesame oil
- 1 tbsp./15ml rice vinegar
- ¼ cup/40g sesame seeds
- ½ cup/60g sliced carrots
- ½ cup/60g zucchini, thinly sliced
- Salt and pepper to taste

Instructions:

1. Heat the garlic-infused olive oil in a skillet set to medium heat.
2. Add the chicken slices and cook for 5-6 minutes until browned and cooked through.
3. Add the sesame oil, rice vinegar, and sliced vegetables (carrots and zucchini). Stir-fry for another 3-4 minutes.
4. Sprinkle using sesame seeds then season with salt and pepper.
5. Serve in bowls then garnish with fresh cilantro or green onions if desired.
6. Pair with your favorite low-FODMAP side dishes.

Per serving:

Calories: 370kcal | Fat: 20g | Carbs: 10g | Protein: 28g | Fiber: 4g | Sugar: 6g

MAIN DISHES

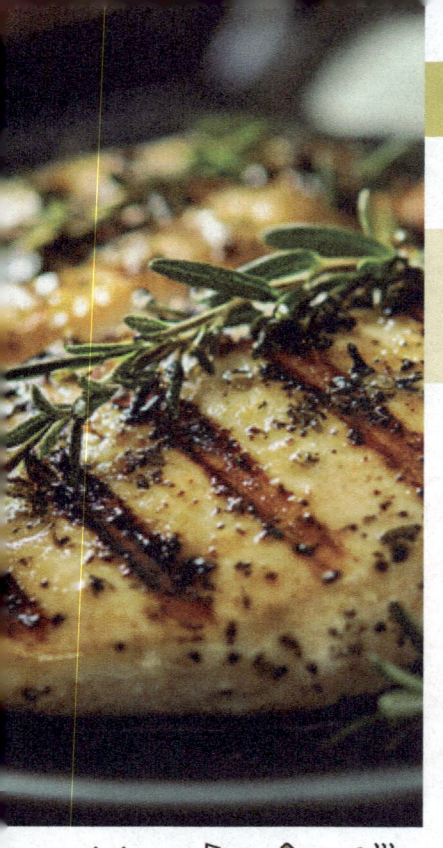

HERB-GRILLED CHICKEN BREAST

Ingredients:

- 2 chicken breasts, boneless and skinless
- 1 tbsp. olive oil
- 1 tsp. fresh thyme, chopped
- 1 tbsp. olive oil
- 1 tsp. fresh rosemary, chopped
- Salt and pepper to taste

Instructions:

1. Preheat a grill pan over medium-high heat.
2. In a small bowl, combine chopped thyme, olive oil, rosemary, salt, and pepper.
3. Rub the mixture equally onto the chicken breasts.
4. Grill the chicken for 6-7 minutes per side, or until the internal temperature reaches 165°F/74°C and the juices run clear.
5. Serve immediately with a side of low-FODMAP vegetables or a light salad (refer to recipes in the previous chapter).

Medium | 2 Servings | 5 min | 15-20 min

Per serving:
Calories: 250 kcal | Fat: 12g | Carbs: 0g | Protein: 26g | Fiber: 0g | Sugar: 0g

Medium | 2 Servings | 10 min | 5 min

ZUCCHINI NOODLES WITH PESTO SAUCE

Ingredients:

- 2 medium zucchinis, spiralized into noodles
- Salt and pepper to taste
- ¾ cup/180ml Fresh Herb Pesto Sauce (see recipe p.67)

Instructions:

1. Heat a skillet set to medium heat then sauté zucchini noodles for 2-3 minutes until just tender.
2. Toss the noodles with the pesto sauce, adding salt and pepper to taste.
3. Serve warm as a light main dish and pair it with your favorite low-FODMAP side dishes.

Per serving:
Calories: 300kcal | Fat: 18g | Carbs: 14g | Protein: 5g | Fiber: 3g | Sugar: 5g

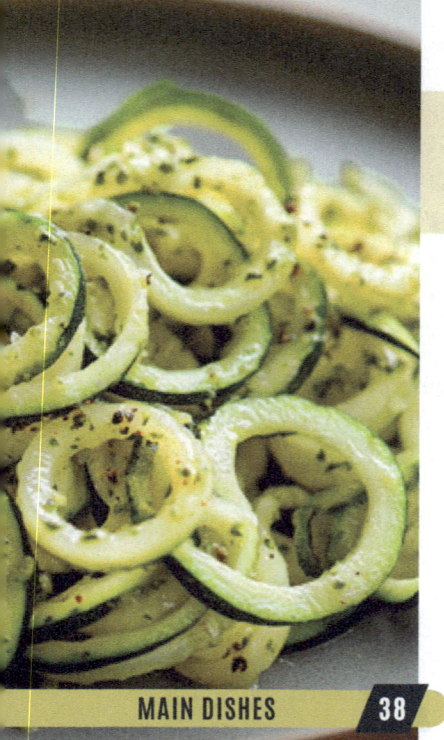

MAIN DISHES

THAI BASIL CHICKEN STIR-FRY

Ingredients:

- 2 chicken breasts, thinly sliced
- 1 tbsp. Garlic-Infused Olive Oil (see recipe p.70)
- ½ green bell pepper, thinly sliced
- 1 tbsp./15ml fish sauce (ensure gluten-free)
- 1 tsp. fresh basil, chopped
- ½ zucchini, thinly sliced
- Salt and pepper to taste

Instructions:

1. Heat garlic-infused olive oil in a skillet set to medium heat.
2. Add the sliced chicken and cook for 5-6 minutes, until the chicken is cooked through.
3. Add the bell pepper, zucchini, and fish sauce, stirring until the vegetables are tender.
4. Stir in the fresh basil, season with salt and pepper, then cook for another 2 minutes.
5. Serve immediately with a side of rice, steamed vegetables or salad (refer to recipes in the previous chapter).

Per serving:
Calories: 280 kcal | Fat: 12g | Carbs: 5g | Protein: 28g | Fiber: 2g | Sugar: 3g

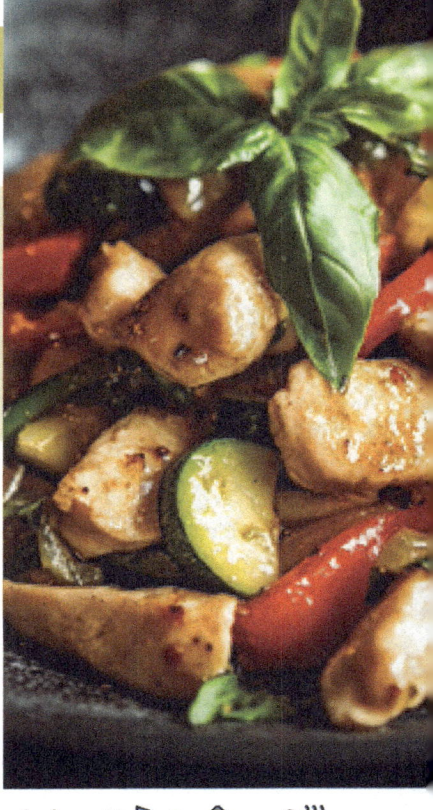

Medium | 2 Servings | 10 min | 10 min

MOROCCAN SPICED FISH TAGINE

Easy | 2 Servings | 10 min | 15-20 min

Ingredients:

- 2 white fish fillets (such as cod or tilapia)
- 1 tbsp. Garlic-Infused Olive Oil (see recipe p.70)
- 1 tbsp. ground cumin
- 1 tbsp. ground coriander
- 1 tsp. ground turmeric
- 1 tsp. paprika
- 1 tbsp./15ml lemon juice
- ½ cup/80g diced tomatoes (fresh)
- Salt and pepper to taste

Instructions:

1. Heat the garlic-infused olive oil in a skillet set to medium heat.
2. Add the cumin, coriander, turmeric, paprika, salt, and pepper to the pan, cooking for 1-2 minutes until fragrant.
3. Bring the fish fillets to the skillet and sear for 2-3 minutes on each side. Stir in the diced tomatoes and lemon juice.
4. Cover and simmer for 15-20 minutes, until the fish is cooked through and flaky. Serve with rice or quinoa.
5. Pair with your favorite low-FODMAP side dishes.

Per serving:
Calories: 300kcal | Fat: 14g | Carbs: 12g | Protein: 28g | Fiber: 3g | Sugar: 4g

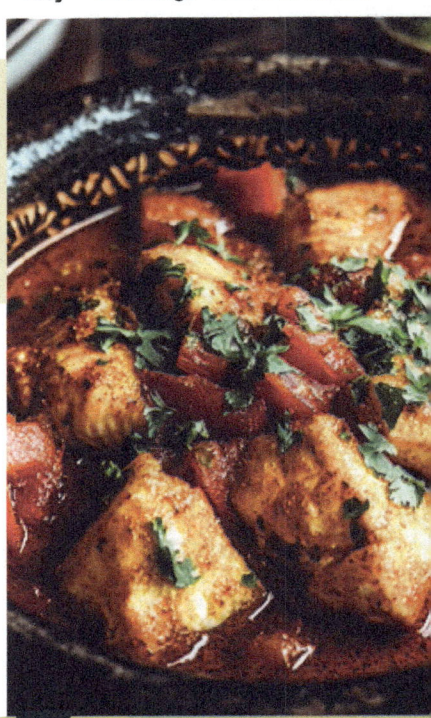

MAIN DISHES

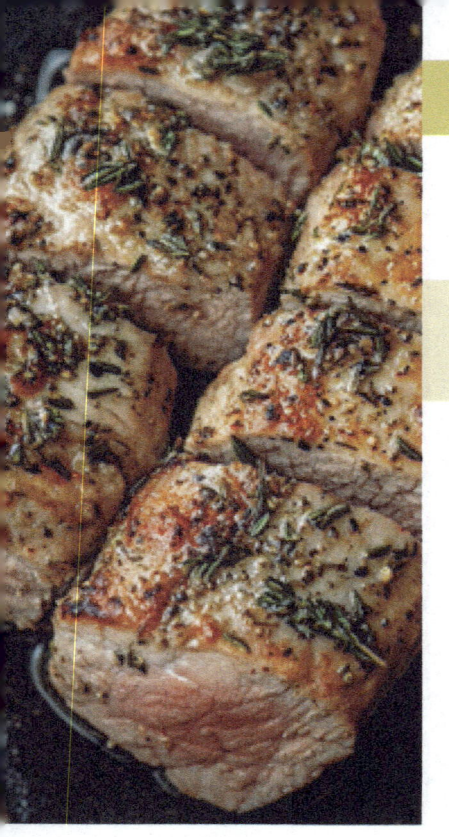

GRILLED PORK WITH HERBS

Ingredients:

- 1 pork tenderloin
- 1 tbsp. Garlic-Infused Olive Oil (see recipe p.70)
- 1 tsp. dried rosemary
- 1 tsp. dried thyme
- Salt and pepper to taste

Instructions:

1. Preheat the grill to medium-high heat.
2. Rub the pork tenderloin with garlic-infused olive oil, rosemary, thyme, salt, and pepper.
3. Grill the pork tenderloin for 10-12 minutes per side or until the internal temperature reaches 145°F/63°C.
4. Remove the pork from the grill then let rest for 5 minutes before slicing.
5. Serve with your favorite low-FODMAP side dishes.

Medium | 2 Servings | 15 min | 20-25 min

Per serving:
Calories: 350 kcal | Fat: 15g | Carbs: 2g | Protein: 38g | Fiber: 0g | Sugar: 1g

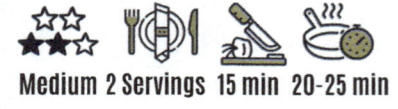

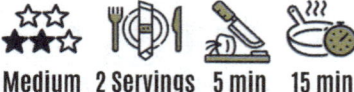

BAKED TILAPIA WITH DILL SAUCE

Medium | 2 Servings | 5 min | 15 min

Ingredients:

- 2 tilapia fillets
- 1 tbsp. olive oil
- Salt and pepper to taste
- 1 tbsp. fresh dill, chopped
- ½ cup/120g lactose-free sour cream
- 1 tsp./5ml lemon juice

Instructions:

1. Preheat the oven to 375°F/190°C.
2. Arrange the tilapia fillets on a baking sheet lined with parchment paper. Drizzle the fillets using olive oil and season with salt and pepper.
3. Bake for 12-15 minutes, or until the fish easily flakes when tested with a fork. In a small bowl, mix the lactose-free sour cream, fresh dill, and lemon juice to create the dill sauce.
4. Serve the baked tilapia topped with the dill sauce.
5. Pair with your favorite low-FODMAP side dishes.

Per serving:
Calories: 300 kcal | Fat: 14g | Carbs: 6g | Protein: 26g | Fiber: 1g | Sugar: 2g

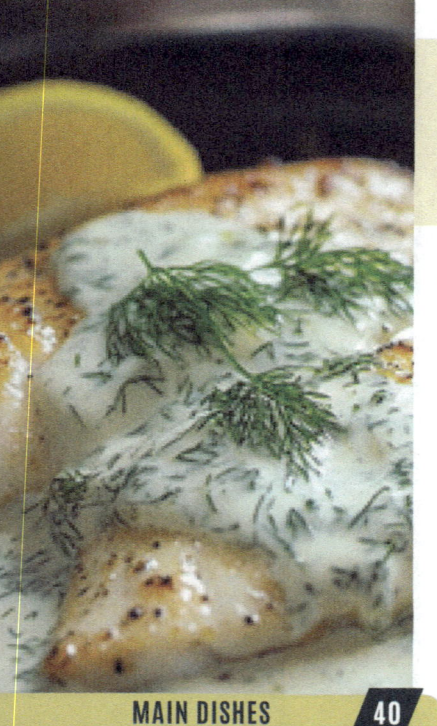

MAIN DISHES

EGGPLANT RATATOUILLE

Ingredients:

- 1 medium eggplant, diced
- 1 zucchini, diced
- 1 green bell pepper, diced
- ½ cup/80g diced tomatoes (fresh)
- 1 tbsp. Garlic-Infused Olive Oil (see recipe p.70)
- 1 tsp. dried oregano
- 1 tsp. dried basil
- Salt and pepper to taste

Instructions:

1. Heat the garlic-infused olive oil in a large skillet set to medium heat.
2. Add the eggplant, zucchini, and bell pepper, cooking for 10-12 minutes until softened.
3. Stir in the basil, diced tomatoes, oregano, salt, and pepper, and cook for an additional 10-12 minutes until the vegetables are tender and the sauce thickens.
4. Serve hot and pair it with your favorite low-FODMAP side dishes.

Per serving:
Calories: 230 kcal | Fat: 12g | Carbs: 18g | Protein: 3g | Fiber: 6g | Sugar: 8g

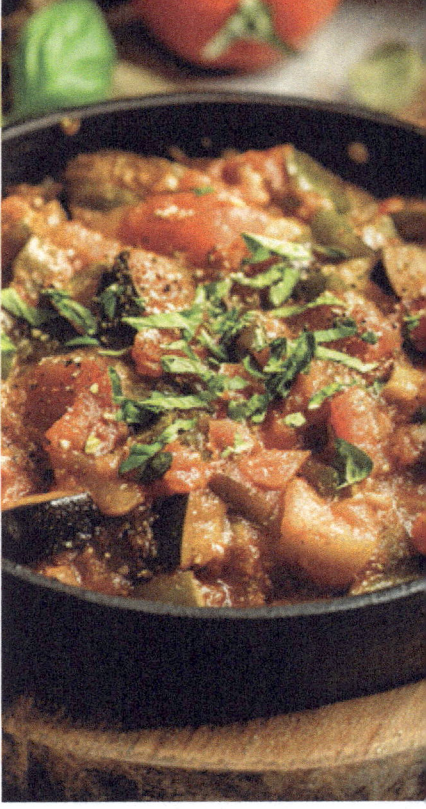

Medium | 2 Servings | 15 min | 30 min

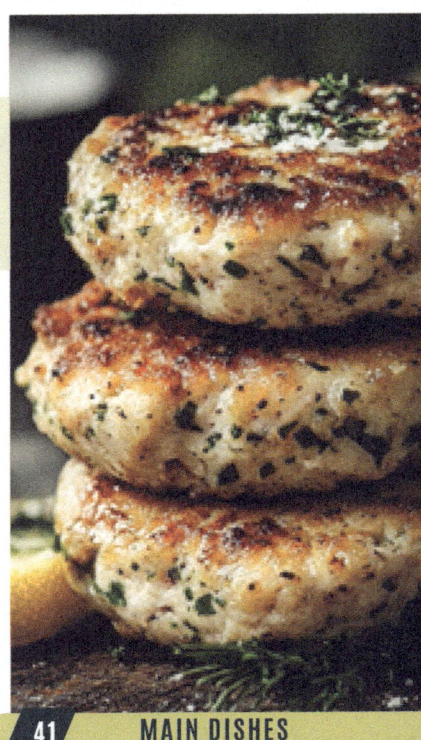

LEMON AND HERB TURKEY PATTIES

Medium | 2 Servings | 10 min | 10-12 min

Ingredients:

- 1 lb./450g ground turkey
- 1 tbsp. fresh parsley, chopped
- 1 tbsp. fresh thyme, chopped
- 1 tbsp./6g lemon zest
- 1 tbsp. Garlic-Infused Olive Oil (see recipe 70)
- Salt and pepper to taste

Instructions:

1. In your bowl, combine the ground turkey, parsley, thyme, lemon zest, garlic-infused olive oil, salt, and pepper.
2. Form the mixture into 4 small patties.
3. Heat a skillet set to medium heat then cook the patties for 5-6 minutes on each side, until fully cooked and browned.
4. Serve with a side salad or steamed vegetables (refer to recipes in the previous chapter).

Per serving:
Calories: 300 kcal | Fat: 14g | Carbs: 2g | Protein: 30g | Fiber: 0g | Sugar: 1g

MAIN DISHES

CHICKEN COCONUT CURRY

Ingredients:

- 1 lb./450g chicken breast, cubed
- 1 cup/240ml coconut milk (canned or fresh)
- 1 green bell pepper, sliced
- 1 medium zucchini, sliced
- 1 carrot, thinly sliced
- 1 tbsp. ginger, grated
- 1 tbsp. Garlic-Infused Olive Oil (see recipe p.70)
- 1 tsp. curry powder
- Salt and pepper to taste

Instructions:

1. Heat the garlic-infused olive oil in a large skillet set to medium heat.
2. Add the chicken breast cubes and cook for 5-6 minutes, until browned on all sides.
3. Add the ginger, curry powder, bell pepper, zucchini, and carrot to the pan and cook for another 5 minutes.
4. Drizzle the coconut milk, bring to a simmer, then cook for 10-15 minutes, allowing the sauce to thicken and the vegetables to soften. Season using salt and pepper and serve over rice or quinoa and pair it with your favorite low-FODMAP side dishes.

Per serving:
Calories: 450kcal | Fat: 24g | Carbs: 12g | Protein: 30g | Fiber: 4g | Sugar: 7g

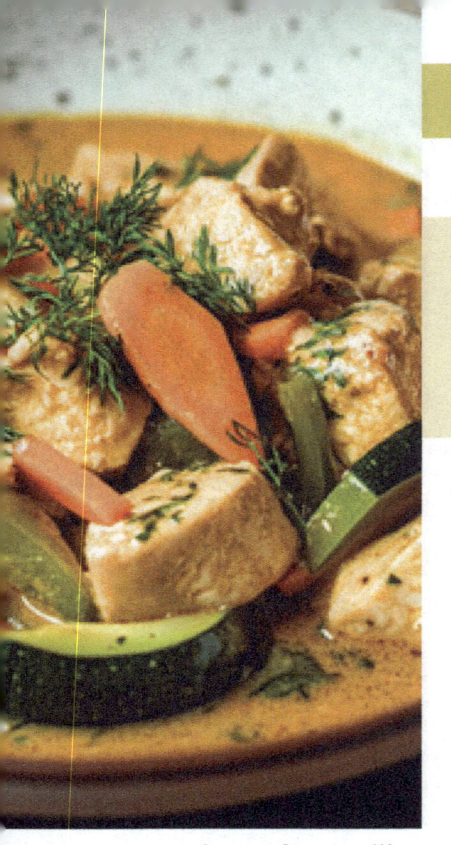

Medium 2 Servings 15 min 25 min

Medium 2 Servings 10 min 30-35min

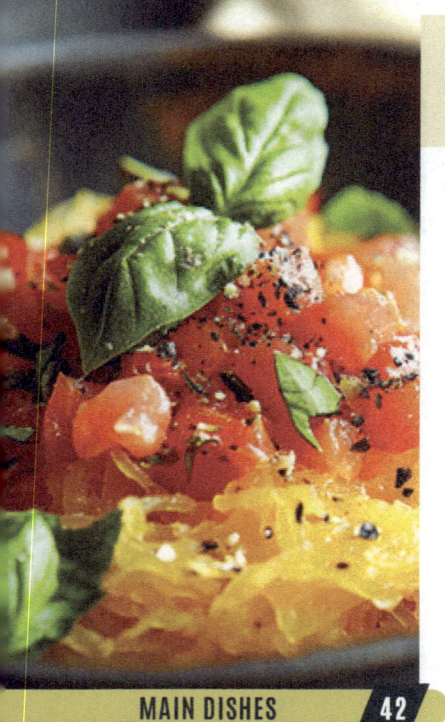

TOMATO BASIL SPAGHETTI SQUASH

Ingredients:

- 1 small spaghetti squash
- 2 medium tomatoes, diced
- 1 tbsp. fresh basil, chopped
- 1 tbsp. Garlic-Infused Olive Oil (see recipe p.70)
- Salt and pepper to taste

Instructions:

1. Preheat the oven to 375°F/190°C. Cut the spaghetti squash in half lengthwise then scoop out the seeds.
2. Drizzle the inside of the squash with garlic-infused olive oil, season using salt and pepper, and place cut-side down on a baking sheet. Roast for 30-35 minutes, until the flesh can be scraped into strands.
3. In a skillet, heat the garlic-infused olive oil set to medium heat. Add the diced tomatoes and cook for 5-6 minutes until softened.
4. Fluff the spaghetti squash strands with a fork and top using the tomato mixture and fresh basil. Serve hot and pair it with your favorite low-FODMAP side dishes.

Per serving:
Calories: 230 kcal | Fat: 12g | Carbs: 18g | Protein: 3g | Fiber: 6g | Sugar: 7g

MAIN DISHES

ROASTED CHICKEN DRUMSTICKS

Ingredients:

- 4 chicken drumsticks
- 1 tbsp. fresh rosemary, chopped
- 2 tbsps. olive oil
- 1 tsp. smoked paprika
- Salt and pepper to taste

Instructions:

1. Preheat the oven to 400°F/200°C.
2. Rub the chicken drumsticks with olive oil, rosemary, smoked paprika, salt, and pepper.
3. Bring the drumsticks on a baking sheet lined with parchment paper.
4. Roast for 40-45 minutes, turning once halfway through, until the drumsticks are golden brown then the internal temperature reaches 165°F/74°C.
5. Serve with roasted vegetables or a side salad (refer to recipes in the previous chapter).

Per serving:
Calories: 370 kcal | Fat: 22g | Carbs: 0g | Protein: 28g | Fiber: 0g | Sugar: 0g

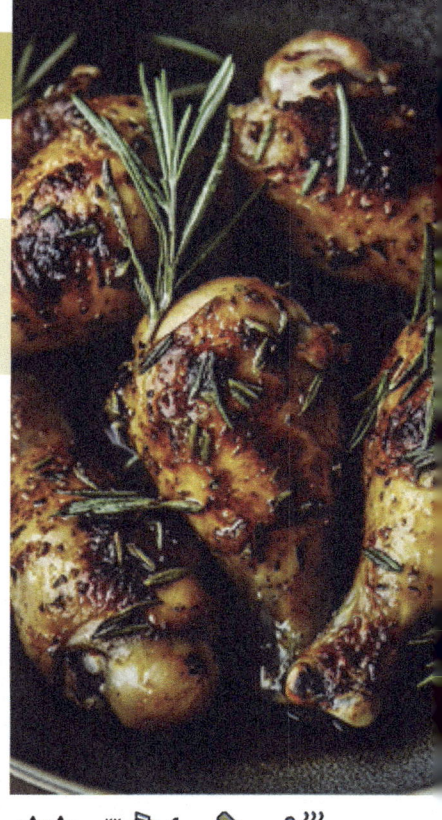

Medium 2 Servings 10 min 40-45 min

BEEF KEBABS WITH VEGGIES

Medium 2 Servings 15 min 12-15 min

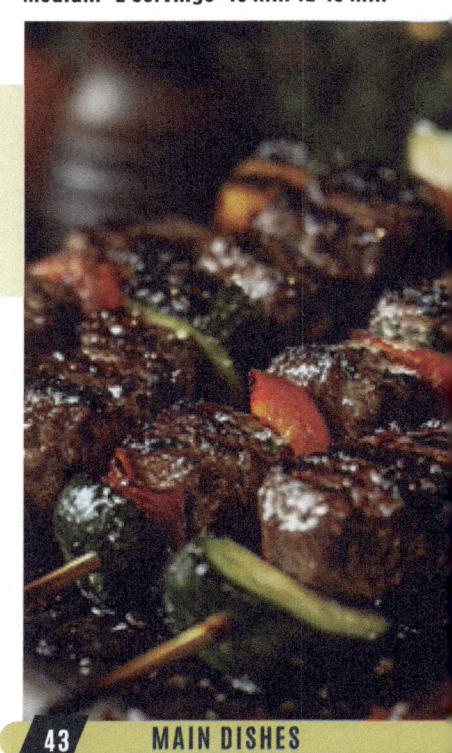

Ingredients:

- 1 lb./450g beef sirloin, cut into 1-inch cubes
- 1 zucchini, sliced
- 1 green bell pepper, cut into chunks
- 1 tbsp. Garlic-Infused Olive Oil (see recipe p.70)
- 1 tbsp. fresh rosemary, chopped
- Salt and pepper to taste

Instructions:

1. Preheat the grill or broiler set to medium-high heat.
2. Thread the beef cubes, zucchini slices, and bell pepper chunks onto skewers.
3. Brush using garlic-infused olive oil and sprinkle with rosemary, salt, and pepper.
4. Grill the kebabs for 12-15 minutes, turning occasionally, until the beef is browned then cooked to your desired level of doneness.
5. Serve with a side of a fresh salad (refer to recipes in the previous chapter).

Per serving:
Calories: 330 kcal | Fat: 16g | Carbs: 10g | Protein: 28g | Fiber: 3g | Sugar: 6g

MAIN DISHES

PAN-SEARED SCALLOPS WITH LEMON

Ingredients:

- 8–10 large scallops
- 1 tbsp. Garlic-Infused Olive Oil (see recipe p.70)
- 1 tbsp./2g fresh lemon zest
- Salt and pepper to taste
- 1 tbsp. fresh parsley, chopped (for garnish)

Instructions:

1. Heat a skillet set to medium-high heat and add the garlic-infused olive oil.
2. Season the scallops with salt and pepper.
3. Once the oil is hot, bring the scallops in the skillet and sear them for about 2-3 minutes on each side, until golden brown and cooked through.
4. Remove the scallops from the skillet and sprinkle with fresh lemon zest and parsley.
5. Serve with a side of steamed vegetables or salad (refer to recipes in the previous chapter).

Per serving:
Calories: 230 kcal | Fat: 8g | Carbs: 4g | Protein: 22g | Fiber: 1g | Sugar: 2g

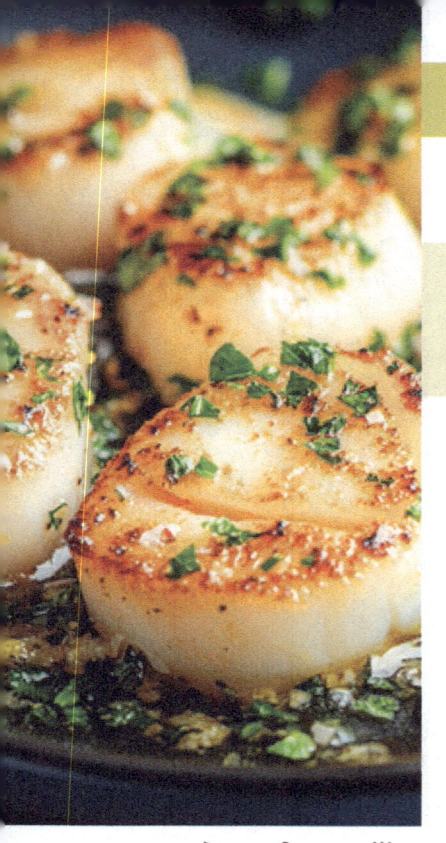

Medium | 2 Servings | 10 min | 15 min

BBQ-STYLE CHICKEN THIGHS

Medium | 2 Servings | 10 min | 20 min

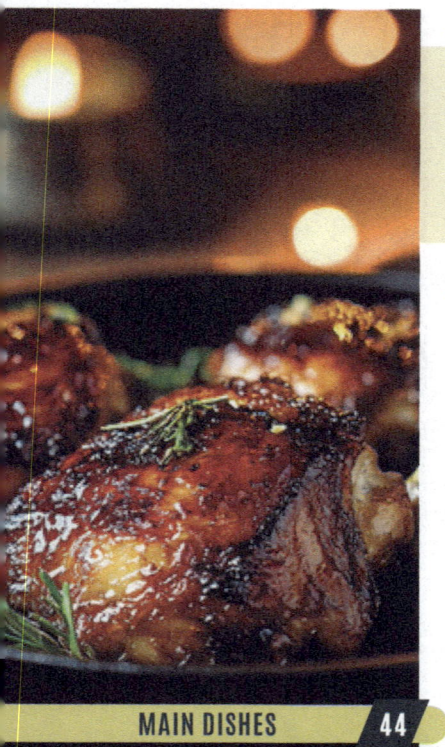

Ingredients:

- 4 chicken thighs, skin-on and bone-in
- 2 tbsps. Garlic-Infused Olive Oil (see recipe p.70)
- 2 tbsps./30ml maple syrup
- 2 tbsps./30ml apple cider vinegar
- 1 tbsp. smoked paprika
- Salt and pepper to taste

Instructions:

1. Preheat the grill or oven set to medium-high heat.
2. In your bowl, mix the garlic-infused olive oil, maple syrup, apple cider vinegar, smoked paprika, salt, and pepper.
3. Coat the chicken thighs with the BBQ marinade and let them sit for at least 10 minutes.
4. Grill the chicken thighs for 8-10 minutes per side, until fully cooked and the skin is crispy.
5. Serve hot with a side salad or roasted vegetables (refer to recipes in the previous chapter).

Per serving:
Calories: 370 kcal | Fat: 22g | Carbs: 10g | Protein: 28g | Fiber: 2g | Sugar: 8g

MAIN DISHES

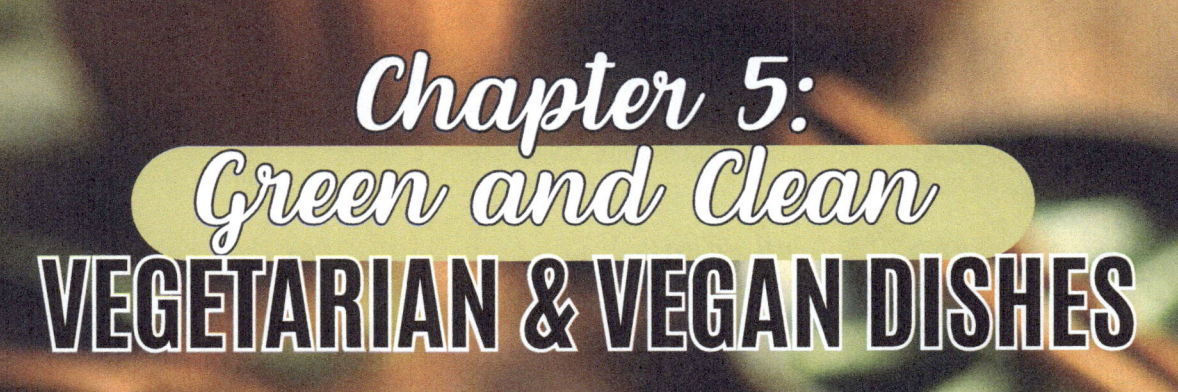

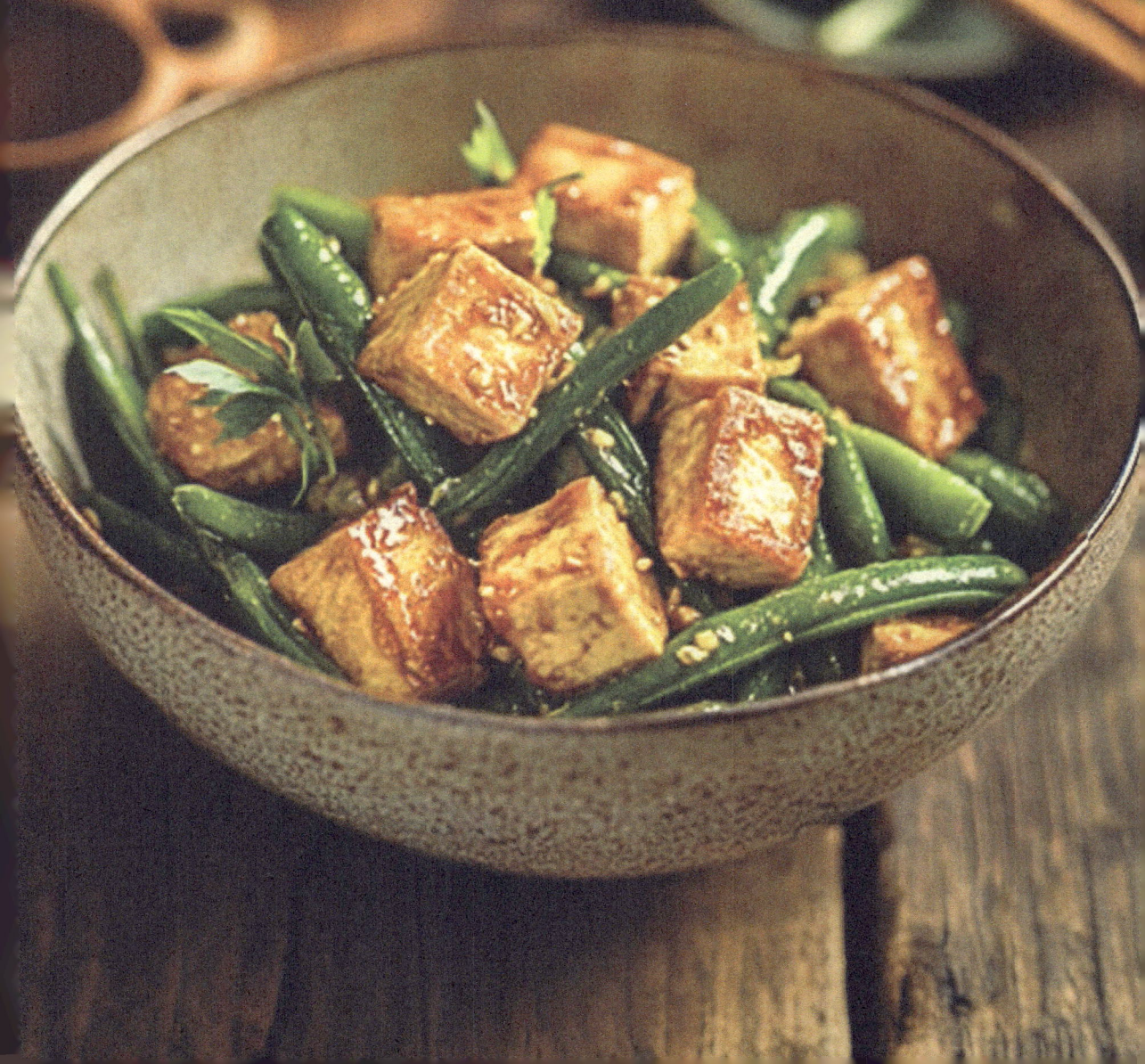

Chapter 5: Green and Clean
VEGETARIAN & VEGAN DISHES

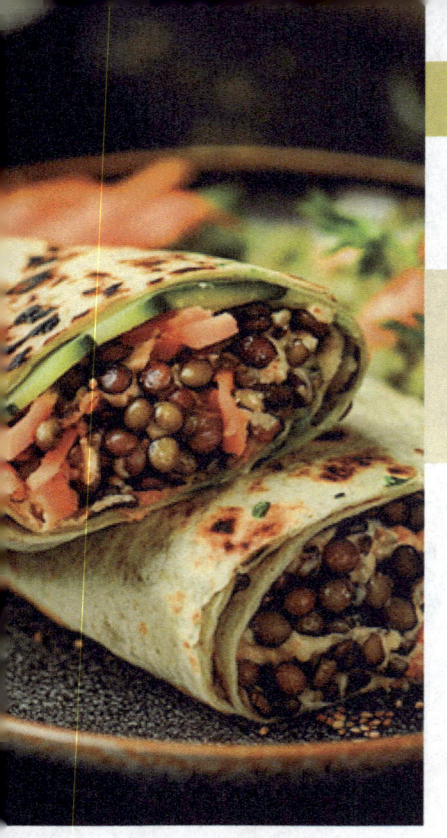

CHICKPEA-FREE HUMMUS WRAP

Ingredients:

- ½ cup/85g cooked lentils
- ½ cup/60g cucumber, sliced
- ¼ cup/30g shredded carrots
- 2 tbsps./30g Hamemade Tahini (see recipe p.66)
- 1 tbsp./15ml lemon juice
- 1 tbsp. olive oil
- 2 gluten-free wraps
- Salt and pepper to taste

Instructions:

1. In a small bowl, mix tahini, olive oil, lemon juice, salt, and pepper to make the hummus.
2. Spread the tahini mixture evenly on the gluten-free wraps.
3. Top with cooked lentils, sliced cucumber, and shredded carrots.
4. Roll the wraps tightly then slice in half.
5. Serve immediately.

Easy | 2 Servings | 10 min | 15 min

Per serving:
Calories: 400 kcal | Fat: 18g | Carbs: 35g | Protein: 10g | Fiber: 8g | Sugar: 4g

Medium | 2 Servings | 15 min | 45 min

VEGAN SHEPHERD'S PIE

Ingredients:

- 2 large sweet potatoes, peeled and cubed
- 1 tbsp. Garlic-Infused Olive Oil (see recipe p.70)
- 1 cup/180g zucchini, diced
- ½ cup/80g carrots, diced
- ½ cup/75g peas
- 1 cup/200g cooked lentils
- 1 tbsp. fresh thyme, chopped
- Salt and pepper to taste
- ¼ cup/60ml Homemade Vegetable Broth (see recipe p.67)

Instructions:

1. Preheat the oven to 375°F/190°C.
2. Boil the sweet potatoes in a large pot of water until tender, about 15 minutes. Drain and mash. Set aside.
3. In a skillet, heat the garlic-infused olive oil set to medium heat. Add the zucchini, carrots, and peas. Sauté for 5-7 minutes.
4. Add the cooked lentils, thyme, salt, pepper, and vegetable broth. Stir to combine and cook for another 5 minutes.
5. Transfer the lentil and vegetable mixture to an oven-safe dish, and top with the mashed sweet potatoes.
6. Bake in the preheated oven for 20 minutes, until golden on top.
7. Serve hot.

Per serving:
Calories: 400 kcal | Fat: 8g | Carbs: 50g | Protein: 13g | Fiber: 10g | Sugar: 12g

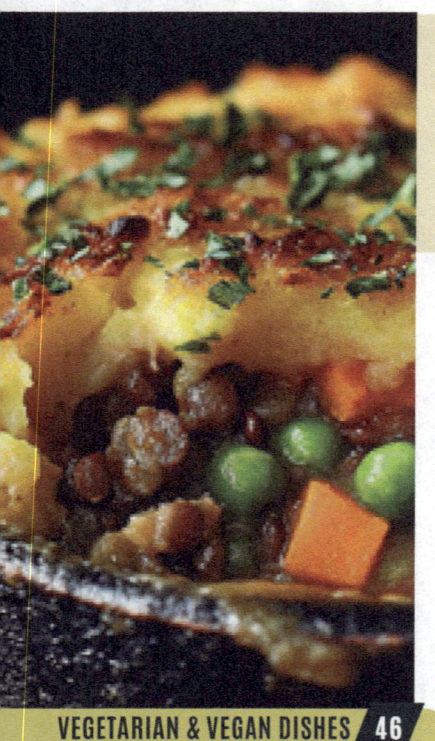

VEGETARIAN & VEGAN DISHES

COCONUT CURRY LENTIL SOUP

Ingredients:

- 1 cup/200g cooked lentils
- 1 tbsp. Garlic-Infused Olive Oil (see recipe p.70)
- 1 tbsp. grated ginger
- 1 tsp. curry powder
- ½ tsp. turmeric
- ½ cup/120ml coconut milk
- 2 cups/480ml Homemade Vegetable Broth (see recipe p.67)
- Salt and pepper to taste

Instructions:

1. Heat the garlic-infused olive oil in a large pot over medium heat.
2. Add the grated ginger and spices, sautéing for 2-3 minutes until fragrant.
3. Stir in the lentils, coconut milk, and vegetable broth, then bring to a boil.
4. Reduce the heat then simmer for 15-20 minutes, letting the soup thicken.
5. Season with salt and pepper to taste.
6. Serve warm with a side of rice or gluten-free bread.

Per serving:
Calories: 380 kcal | Fat: 20g | Carbs: 30g | Protein: 10g | Fiber: 8g | Sugar: 5g

Medium 2 Servings 10 min 25 min

EGGPLANT AND TOMATO CASSEROLE

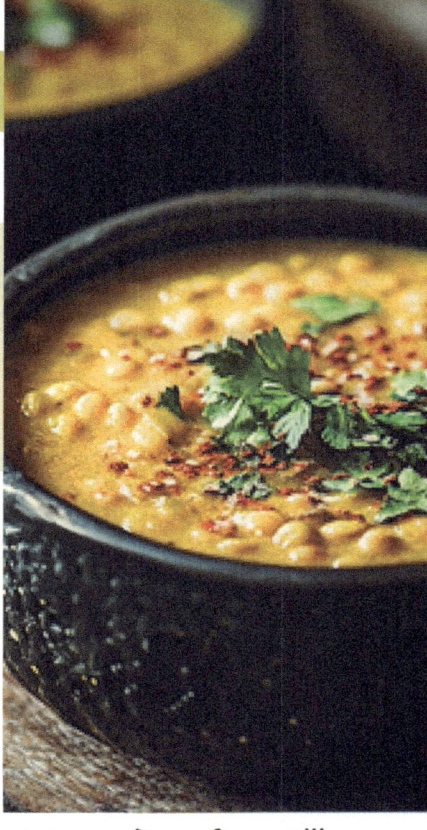

Medium 2 Servings 10 min 40 min

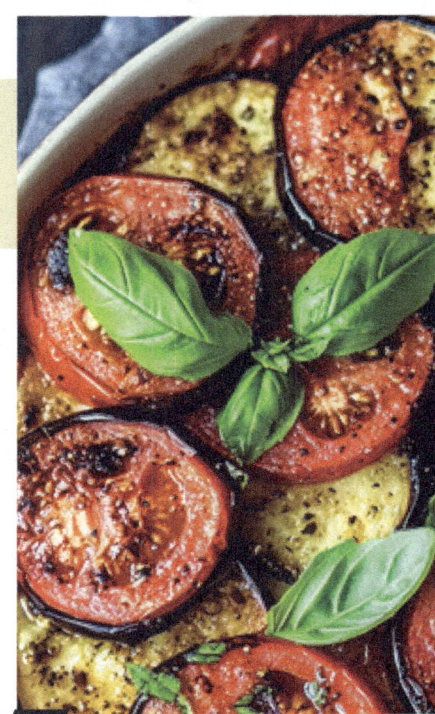

Ingredients:

- 2 medium eggplants, sliced
- 2 tomatoes, diced
- 1 tbsp. ½ tsp. Garlic-Infused Olive Oil (see recipe 70)
- 1 tsp. dried oregano
- 1 tbsp. fresh basil, chopped
- Salt and pepper to taste

Instructions:

1. Preheat the oven to 375°F/190°C.
2. Bring the eggplant slices on a baking sheet, then drizzle with garlic-infused olive oil. Season with salt, pepper, and oregano.
3. Roast the eggplant for 25 minutes, turning the slices halfway through.
4. During the final 10 minutes of roasting, add the diced tomatoes on top of the eggplant and continue baking.
5. Finish with a sprinkle of fresh basil before serving.

Per serving:
Calories: 270 kcal | Fat: 14g | Carbs: 20g | Protein: 4g | Fiber: 7g | Sugar: 8g

VEGETARIAN & VEGAN DISHES

ROASTED VEGETABLE BUDDHA BOWL

Ingredients:

- 1 small sweet potato, cubed
- 1 cup/150g broccoli florets
- ½ cup/60g carrots, thinly sliced
- 1 tbsp. Garlic-Infused Olive Oil (see recipe p.70)
- 1 tbsp. olive oil
- 1 cup/170g cooked quinoa
- 1 tbsp./15g Hamemade Tahini (see recipe p.66)
- 1 tbsp./15ml lemon juice
- Salt and pepper to taste

Instructions:

1. Preheat the oven to 400°F/200°C.
2. Toss the sweet potato, broccoli, and carrots in garlic-infused olive oil, salt, and pepper. Spread them out on a baking sheet.
3. Roast the vegetables for 20-25 minutes, or until tender and lightly browned.
4. In a small bowl, whisk together the tahini, olive oil, lemon juice, salt, and pepper to make the dressing.
5. To assemble, place the cooked quinoa in bowls and top with the roasted vegetables. Drizzle with the tahini dressing.
6. Serve warm or at room temperature.

Per serving:
Calories: 400 kcal | Fat: 18g | Carbs: 40g | Protein: 8g | Fiber: 9g | Sugar: 8g

Medium | 2 Servings | 15 min | 25 min

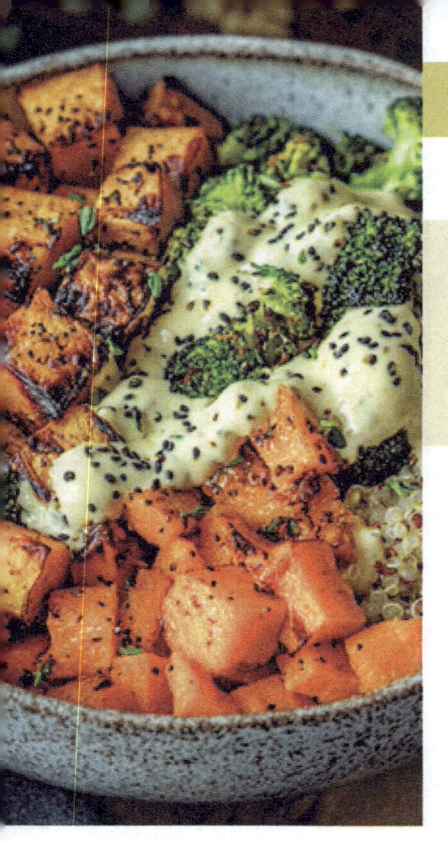

Easy | 2 Servings | 10 min | 30 min

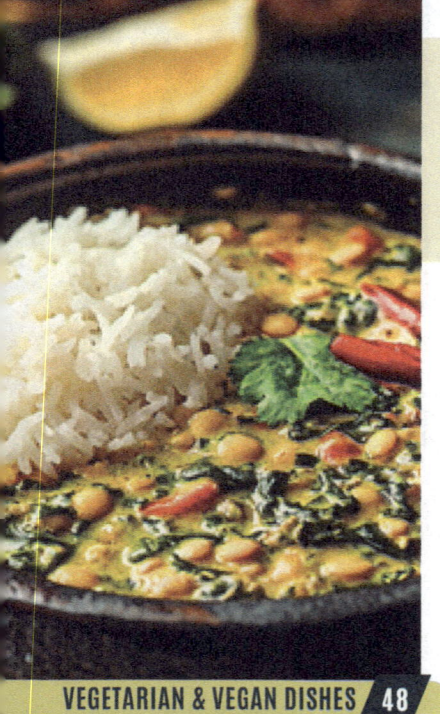

LENTIL AND SPINACH CURRY

Ingredients:

- 1 cup/200g cooked lentils
- 1 cup/30g spinach leaves, fresh
- 1 tbsp. Garlic-Infused Olive Oil (see recipe 70)
- 1 tbsp. fresh ginger, grated
- ½ tsp. turmeric powder
- 1 tsp. ground cumin
- ½ tsp. ground coriander
- ¼ tsp. ground cinnamon
- ½ cup/120ml coconut milk
- Salt and pepper to taste

Instructions:

1. Heat the garlic-infused olive oil in a large pan set to medium heat.
2. Add the grated ginger and spices (turmeric, cumin, coriander, cinnamon) to the pan and sauté for 2 minutes until fragrant.
3. Add the cooked lentils and coconut milk, stirring well to combine.
4. Simmer for 10-15 minutes, allowing the curry to thicken.
5. Add the spinach and cook for extra 2 minutes until wilted.
6. Season using salt and pepper to taste and serve with rice or quinoa.

Per serving:
Calories: 350 kcal | Fat: 14g | Carbs: 35g | Protein: 15g | Fiber: 9g | Sugar: 5g

VEGETARIAN & VEGAN DISHES

TOFU STIR-FRY WITH GREEN BEANS

Ingredients:

- 1 block firm tofu (about 400g), pressed and cubed
- 1 tbsp. garlic-infused olive oil (see recipe p.91)
- 1 cup/125g green beans, trimmed
- 1 tbsp. fresh ginger, grated
- 2 tbsps./30ml tamari sauce (see recipe p.96)
- 1 tbsp./15ml rice vinegar
- Salt and pepper to taste

Instructions:

1. Heat the garlic-infused olive oil in a large skillet over medium-high heat.
2. Add the cubed tofu and sauté until golden brown then crispy on all sides, about 5-7 minutes.
3. Add the green beans and grated ginger, cooking for another 3-4 minutes until the green beans are tender.
4. Stir in the tamari sauce and rice vinegar. Cook for an additional 2 minutes.
5. Season using salt and pepper to taste and serve with a side of steamed rice or quinoa.

Per serving:
Calories: 330kcal | Fat: 16g | Carbs: 15g | Protein: 22g | Fiber: 5g | Sugar: 6g

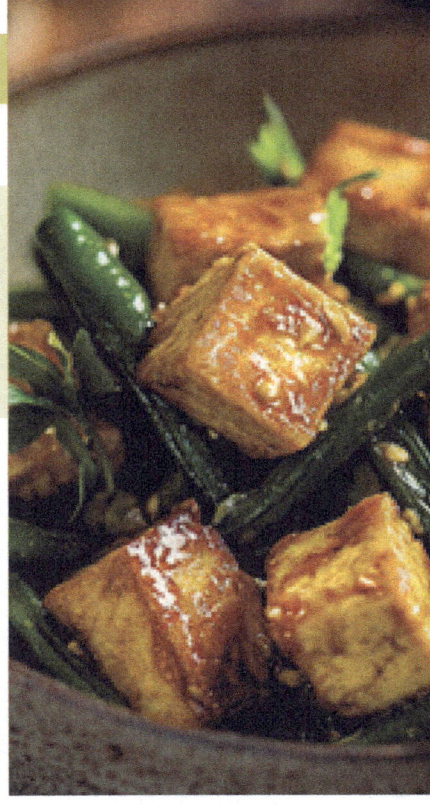

Medium | 2 Servings | 10 min | 15 min

ZUCCHINI LASAGNA WITH RICOTTA

Medium | 2 Servings | 15 min | 35 min

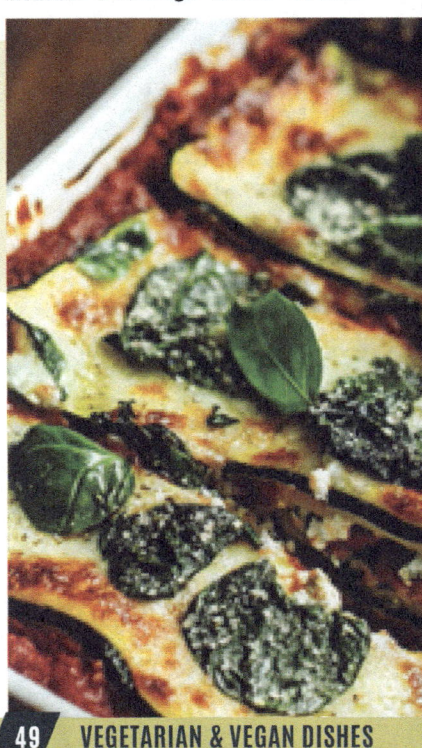

Ingredients:

- 2 medium zucchinis, sliced thinly lengthwise
- 1 cup/240g almond ricotta (made by blending ½ cup almonds, water, and a pinch of salt)
- 1 tbsp. olive oil
- 1 cup/30g fresh spinach, chopped
- ½ cup/120ml Homemade Tomato Sauce (see recipe 66)
- Salt and pepper to taste
- Fresh basil leaves, for garnish

Instructions:

1. Preheat the oven to 375°F/190°C.
2. Heat olive oil in a pan then sauté the spinach until wilted.
3. Spread a thin layer of tomato sauce on the bottom of a baking dish.
4. Layer the zucchini slices, almond ricotta, sautéed spinach, and more tomato sauce. Repeat layers until the ingredients are used up.
5. Cover using foil and bake for 30 minutes.
6. Remove the foil then bake for extra 5 minutes to brown the top.
7. Garnish with fresh basil and serve.

Per serving:
Calories: 340 kcal | Fat: 18g | Carbs: 18g | Protein: 10g | Fiber: 6g | Sugar: 7g

VEGETARIAN & VEGAN DISHES

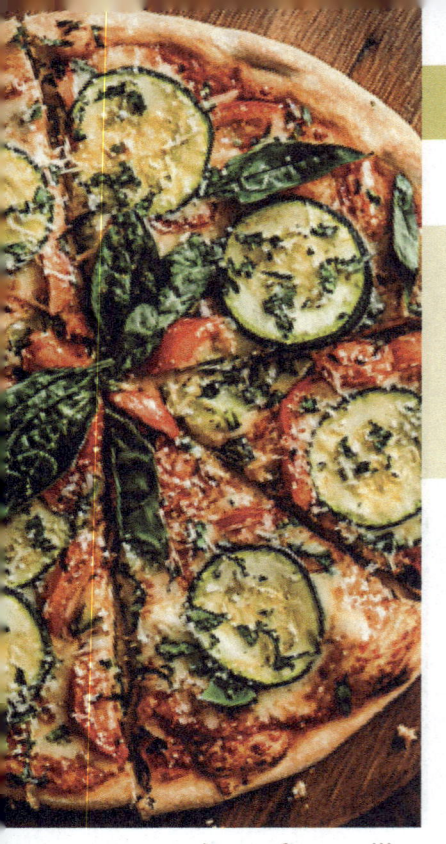

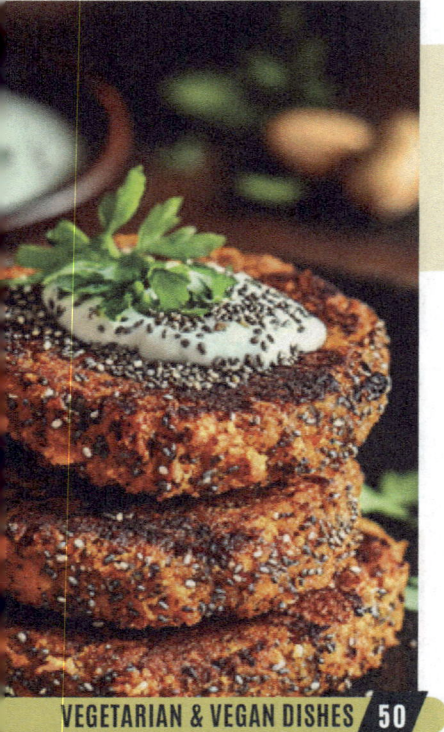

GLUTEN-FREE VEGGIE PIZZA

Ingredients:

- 1 gluten-free pizza base (store-bought or homemade)
- ½ cup/120g Homemade Tomato Sauce (see recipe p.66)
- ½ cup/60g zucchini, sliced
- ¼ cup/30g green bell peppers, sliced
- 1 tbsp. olive oil
- ¼ cup/30g spinach, chopped
- ½ cup/60g lactose-free mozzarella, shredded
- 1 tsp. dried oregano
- Salt and pepper to taste

Instructions:

1. Preheat the oven to 375°F/190°C.
2. Spread the tomato sauce evenly on the gluten-free pizza base.
3. Top with zucchini, bell peppers, and spinach.
4. Sprinkle shredded mozzarella cheese on top.
5. Drizzle with olive oil and sprinkle with dried oregano, salt, and pepper.
6. Bake for 15-20 minutes, or until the crust is crispy and the cheese is melted.
7. Slice and serve.

Medium | 2 Servings | 15 min | 20 min

Per serving:
Calories: 330 kcal | Fat: 14g | Carbs: 30g | Protein: 12g | Fiber: 4g | Sugar: 6g

SWEET POTATO PATTIES

Medium | 2 Servings | 15 min | 20 min

Ingredients:

- 1 large sweet potato, peeled and grated (about 300g)
- ¼ cup/30g gluten-free breadcrumbs
- 1 tbsp. chia seeds (optional)
- ¼ tsp. ground cumin
- Salt and pepper to taste
- ¼ cup/60g coconut yogurt (lactose-free)
- 1 tsp./5ml lemon juice
- Fresh parsley for garnish

Instructions:

1. In a large bowl, mix the grated sweet potato, gluten-free breadcrumbs, chia seeds, cumin, salt, and pepper.
2. Shape the mixture into small patties.
3. Heat a non-stick skillet set to medium heat then cook the patties for 4-5 minutes on each side, or until they are golden and crispy.
4. In a separate small bowl, combine coconut yogurt with lemon juice to create the dip.
5. Serve the sweet potato patties with the coconut yogurt dip, and garnish with fresh parsley.

Per serving:
Calories: 330 kcal | Fat: 12g | Carbs: 38g | Protein: 5g | Fiber: 7g | Sugar: 10g

VEGETARIAN & VEGAN DISHES

Chapter 6: Quick Fueling SNACKS

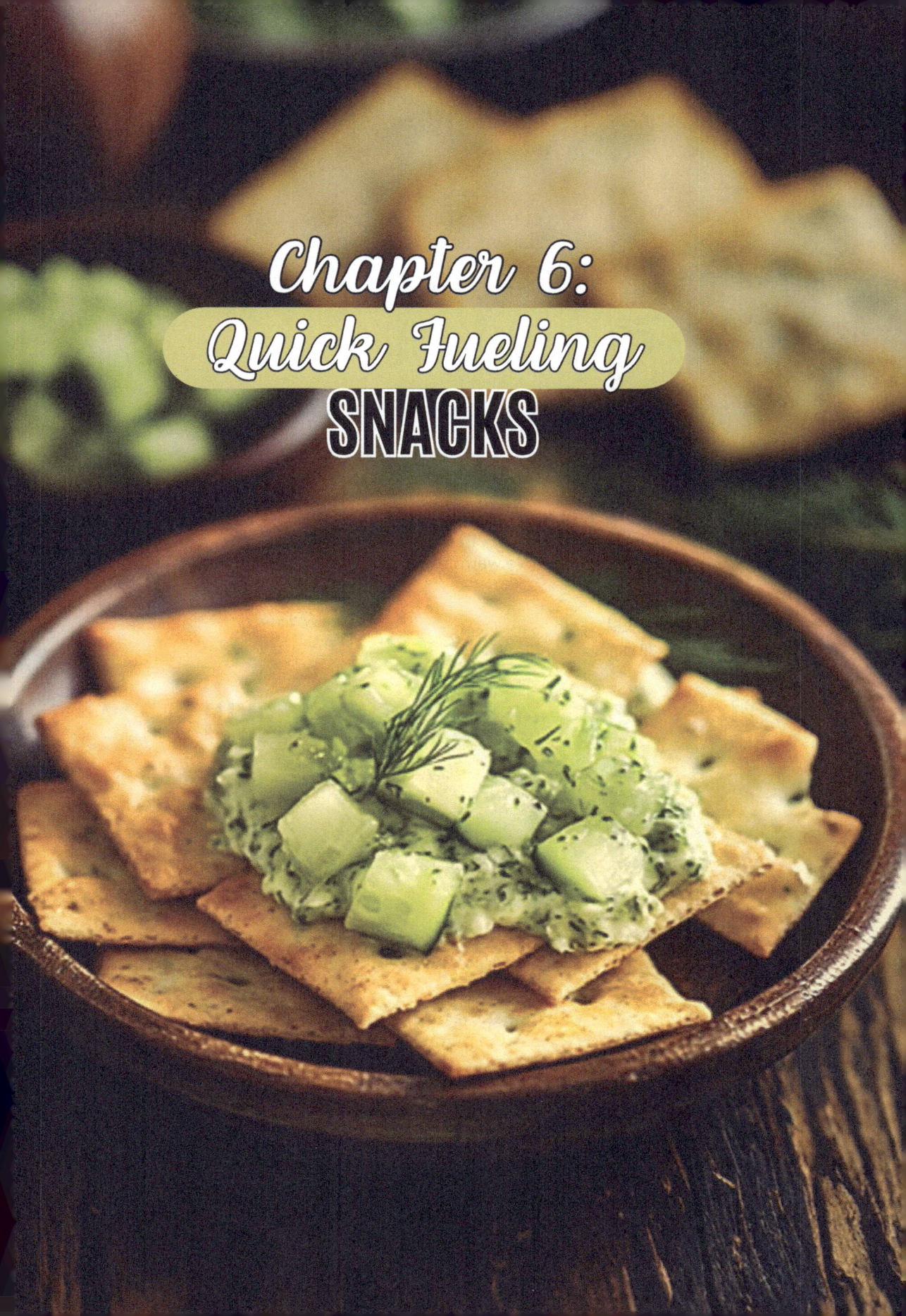

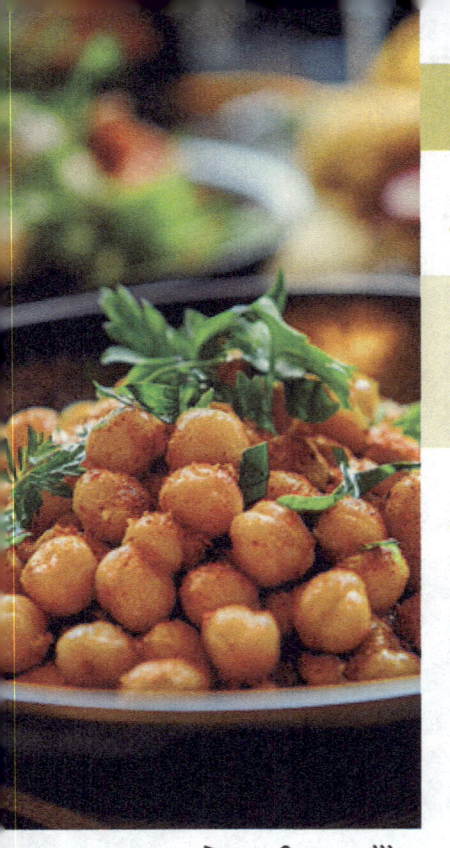

ROASTED CHICKPEAS

Ingredients:

- 1 cup/160g canned chickpeas (drained, rinsed, and patted dry)
- 1 tbsp. olive oil
- ½ tsp. paprika
- ¼ tsp. cumin
- Salt and pepper to taste

Instructions:

1. Preheat the oven to 400°F/200°C.
2. Apply the chickpeas on a baking sheet lined using parchment paper. Drizzle with olive oil then sprinkle using paprika, cumin, salt, and pepper.
3. Toss to coat evenly.
4. Roast in the oven for 25-30 minutes, shaking the pan halfway through, until golden and crispy.
5. Serve warm or, once cooled, store in an airtight container.

Easy | 2 Servings | 10 min | 30 min

Per serving:
Calories: 220 kcal | Fat: 8g | Carbs: 18g | Protein: 7g | Fiber: 5g | Sugar: 2g

ROASTED PUMPKIN SEEDS

Easy | 2 Servings | 5 min | 15-20 min

Ingredients:

- ½ cup/75g pumpkin seeds (raw)
- 1 tbsp. olive oil
- Salt to taste
- ¼ tsp. smoked paprika (optional, for flavor)

Instructions:

1. Preheat the oven to 350°F/180°C.
2. Toss the pumpkin seeds with salt, olive oil, and smoked paprika (if using).
3. Apply the seeds in a single layer on a baking sheet.
4. Roast for 15-20 minutes, stirring halfway through, until they are golden and crispy.
5. Let them cool before serving.

Per serving:
Calories: 210 kcal | Fat: 14g | Carbs: 4g | Protein: 7g | Fiber: 2g | Sugar: 0g

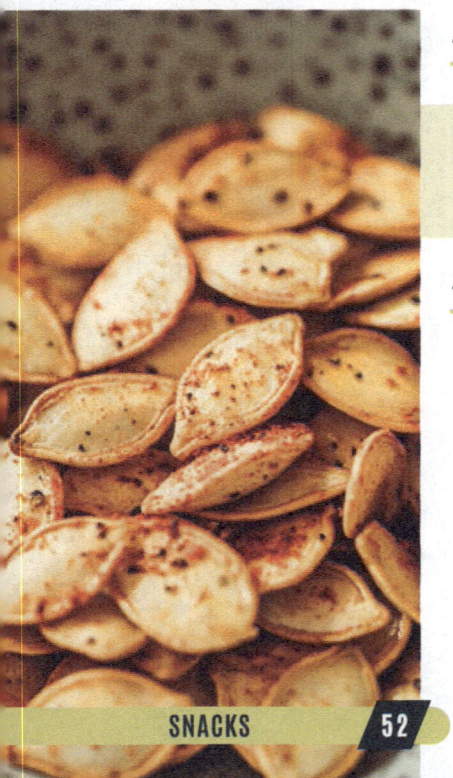

SNACKS

RASPBERRY CHIA JAM

Ingredients:

- ½ cup/75g fresh raspberries (about 20 berries)
- 2 tsps. chia seeds
- 2 tsps./10ml pure maple syrup (optional, adjust to taste)

Instructions:

1. Mash raspberries in a small bowl using a fork until smooth and jam-like.
2. Stir in the chia seeds and maple syrup, ensuring everything is well combined.
3. Let the mixture rest for 10 minutes to let the chia seeds to soften and thicken.
4. Serve as a topping for gluten-free toast, rice cakes, or pair with a side of fresh fruit as a snack. Store any leftovers in an airtight container in the fridge for up to 3 days.

Per serving:
Calories: 95 kcal | Fat: 1g | Carbs: 8g | Protein: 1g | Fiber: 3g | Sugar: 4g

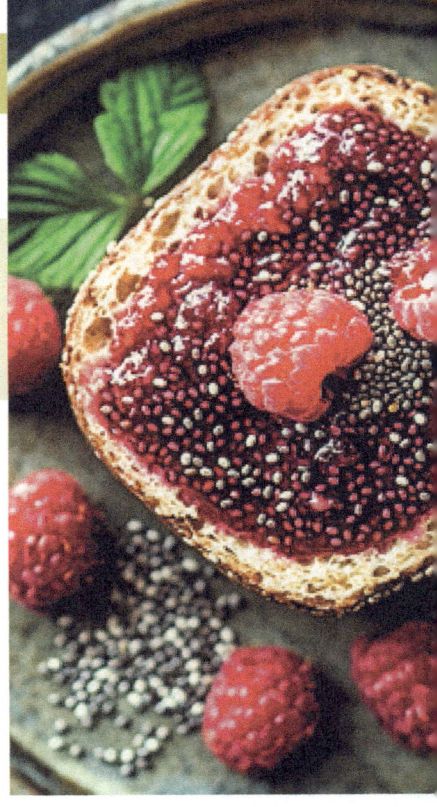

Easy | 2 Servings | 15 min | 0 min

BAKED KALE CHIPS WITH LEMON ZEST

Easy | 2 Servings | 5 min | 15-20min

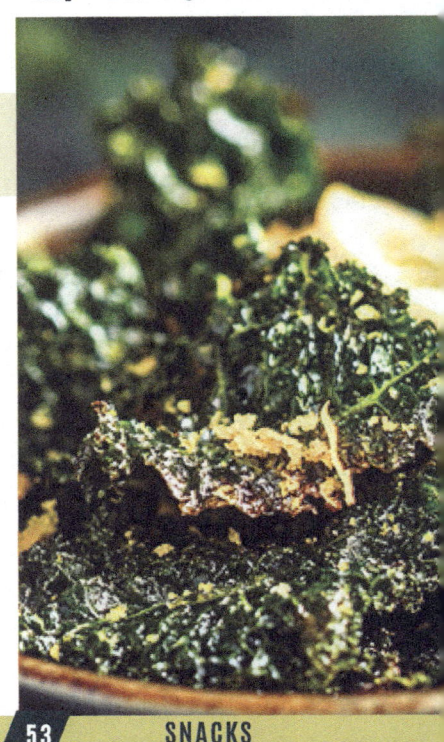

Ingredients:

- 4-5 large kale leaves
- 1 tbsp. olive oil
- ¼ tsp. salt
- Zest of ½ lemon

Instructions:

1. Preheat the oven to 350°F/180°C.
2. Tear the kale into bite-sized pieces, removing the tough stems.
3. Drizzle the kale with olive oil then sprinkle with salt, tossing to coat evenly.
4. Arrange the kale in a single layer on a baking sheet.
5. Bake for 15-20 minutes, checking often to prevent burning, until the kale is crispy.
6. Remove from the oven and top with freshly grated lemon zest. Serve right away.

Per serving:
Calories: 150 kcal | Fat: 8g | Carbs: 8g | Protein: 3g | Fiber: 3g | Sugar: 1g

SNACKS

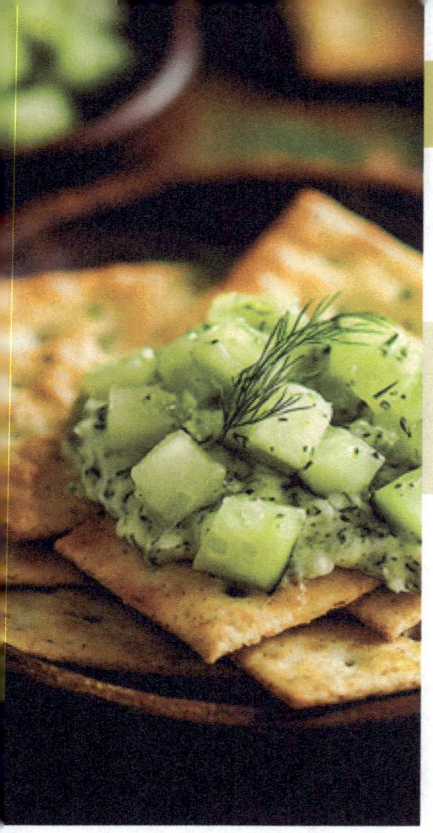

CRACKERS WITH CUCUMBER SPREAD

Ingredients:

- 6-8 gluten-free crackers
- ¼ cucumber/30 g, finely diced
- 1 tbsp. fresh dill, chopped
- Salt and pepper to taste
- 2 tbsps./30g lactose-free cream cheese or dairy-free alternative

Instructions:

1. Mix the diced cucumber, lactose-free cream cheese, dill, salt and pepper in a small bowl.
2. Spread the mixture evenly on the gluten-free crackers.
3. Serve immediately or chill until ready to serve.

Easy | 2 Servings | 10 min | 0 min

Per serving:
Calories: 230 kcal | Fat: 12g | Carbs: 15g | Protein: 4g | Fiber: 2g | Sugar: 2g

CUCUMBER STICKS WITH HUMMUS

Easy | 2 Servings | 10 min | 0 min

Ingredients:

- 1 cucumber, cut into sticks
- ¼ cup/30g pumpkin seeds
- ¼ cup/60g tahini
- 1 tbsp./15ml lemon juice
- 1 tbsp. olive oil
- Salt to taste

Instructions:

1. Place pumpkin seeds, tahini, lemon juice, olive oil, and a pinch of salt in a food processor.
2. Blend until smooth and creamy, adding water to achieve the desired texture if needed.
3. Serve the cucumber sticks with the hummus dip on the side.

Per serving:
Calories: 230 kcal | Fat: 15g | Carbs: 9g | Protein: 6g | Fiber: 3g | Sugar: 3g

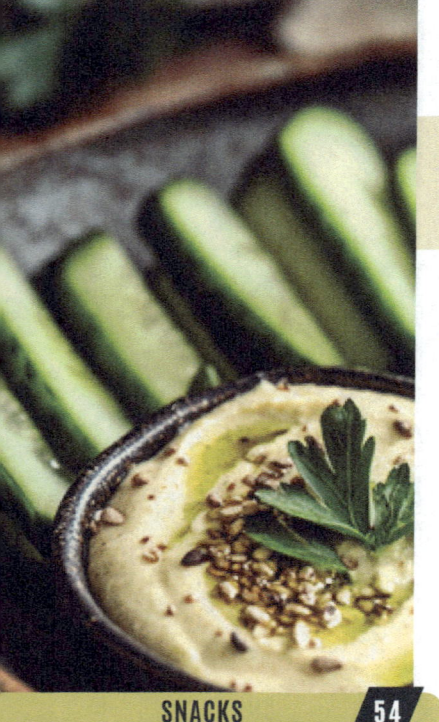

SNACKS

SWEET POTATO CHIPS

Ingredients:

- 1 medium sweet potato, thinly sliced
- 1 tbsp. coconut oil, melted
- Salt to taste
- ¼ tsp. paprika (optional)

Instructions:

1. Preheat your oven to 400°F/200°C.
2. Coat the sweet potato slices with melted coconut oil, salt, and paprika (if desired).
3. Apply the slices in a single layer on a baking sheet lined with parchment paper.
4. Roast for 20-25 minutes, flipping halfway through, until golden and crispy.
5. Serve right away or store in an airtight container for up to 2 days.

Per serving:
Calories: 240 kcal | Fat: 10g | Carbs: 30g | Protein: 2g | Fiber: 4g | Sugar: 6g

Medium 2 Servings 10 min 20-25 min

MINI ZUCCHINI FRITTERS

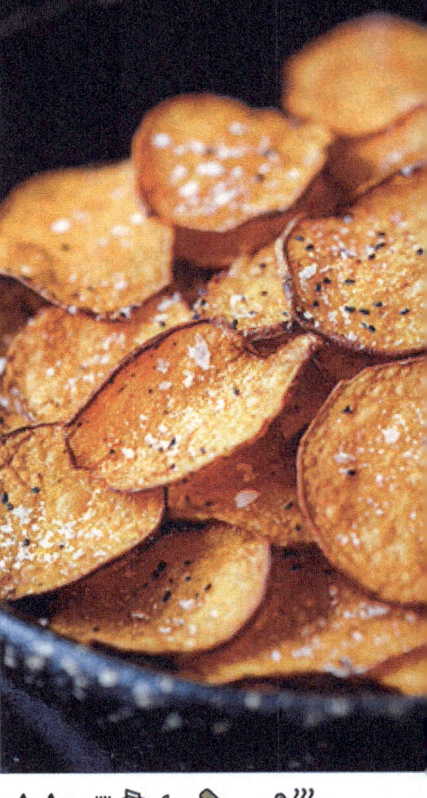

Medium 2 Servings 15 min 10 min

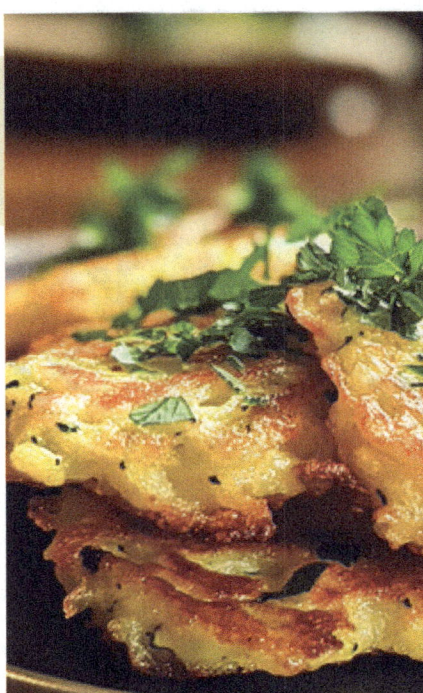

Ingredients:

- 1 medium zucchini, grated
- ¼ cup/30g gluten-free flour
- 1 egg
- 1 tbsp. olive oil
- 1 tbsp. fresh parsley, chopped
- Salt and pepper to taste

Instructions:

1. Grate the zucchini and place it in a clean kitchen towel to squeeze out excess moisture.
2. In your bowl, mix the zucchini, gluten-free flour, egg, parsley, salt, and pepper.
3. Heat olive oil in a non-stick skillet set to medium heat.
4. Scoop a tbsp./15g of the zucchini mixture and flatten it into a fritter shape in the pan.
5. Cook for 2-3 minutes on each side, or until golden and crispy.
6. Serve immediately with a side of low-FODMAP yogurt dip or enjoy on their own.

Per serving:
Calories: 210 kcal | Fat: 10g | Carbs: 14g | Protein: 5g | Fiber: 3g | Sugar: 3g

SNACKS

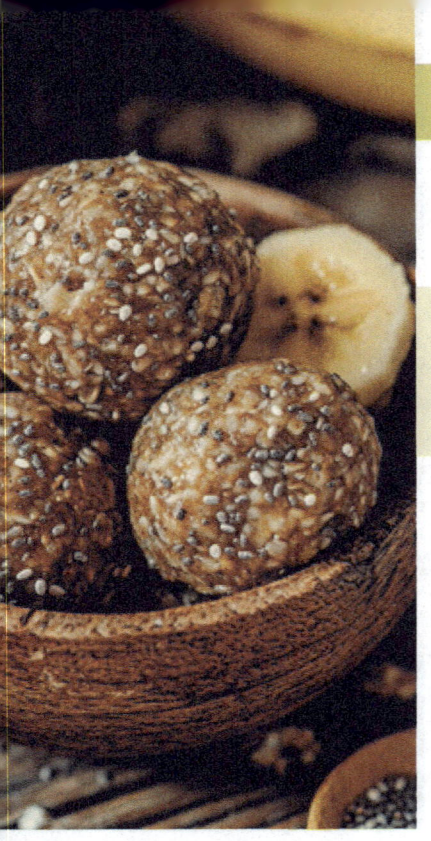

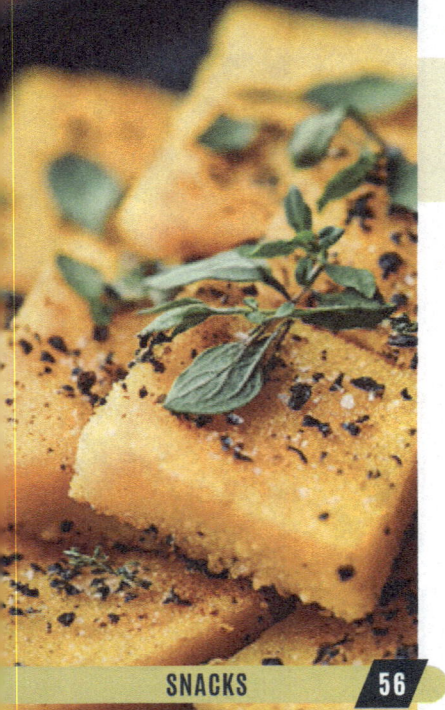

BANANA ENERGY BALLS

Ingredients:

- 1 ripe banana, mashed
- ½ cup/45g gluten-free rolled oats
- 2 tbsps./30g almond butter
- 1 tbsp. chia seeds
- ¼ tsp. ground cinnamon
- 1 tbsp./15g maple syrup (optional)

Instructions:

1. In a mixing bowl, combine mashed banana, oats, almond butter, chia seeds, cinnamon, and maple syrup.
2. Mix until well combined, then shape into small balls (about inch/2.5 cm in diameter).
3. Refrigerate for 15-20 minutes to set.
4. Serve as a quick snack or store in the fridge for later.

Medium | 2 Servings | 15 min | 0 min

Per serving:
Calories: 270 kcal | Fat: 11g | Carbs: 30g | Protein: 5g | Fiber: 4g | Sugar: 12g

Medium | 2 Servings | 10 min | 30 min

BAKED POLENTA SQUARES

Ingredients:

- 1 cup/150g polenta (cornmeal)
- 3 cups/720ml water
- 1 tbsp. olive oil
- ¼ tsp. salt
- ¼ tsp. dried oregano (optional)

Instructions:

1. Preheat the oven up to 375°F/190°C and grease a baking dish.
2. In a saucepan, bring water to a boil. Slowly whisk in the polenta then cook, stirring constantly, for 3-4 minutes until thickened.
3. Stir in olive oil, salt, and oregano.
4. Pour the polenta mixture into the greased baking dish and smooth the top.
5. Bake for 25-30 minutes, until the edges are golden and crispy.
6. Allow it to cool slightly before cutting into squares.

Per serving:
Calories: 230 kcal | Fat: 6g | Carbs: 28g | Protein: 3g | Fiber: 2g | Sugar: 0g

SNACKS

Chapter 7:
WHOLESOME DESSERT
Creations

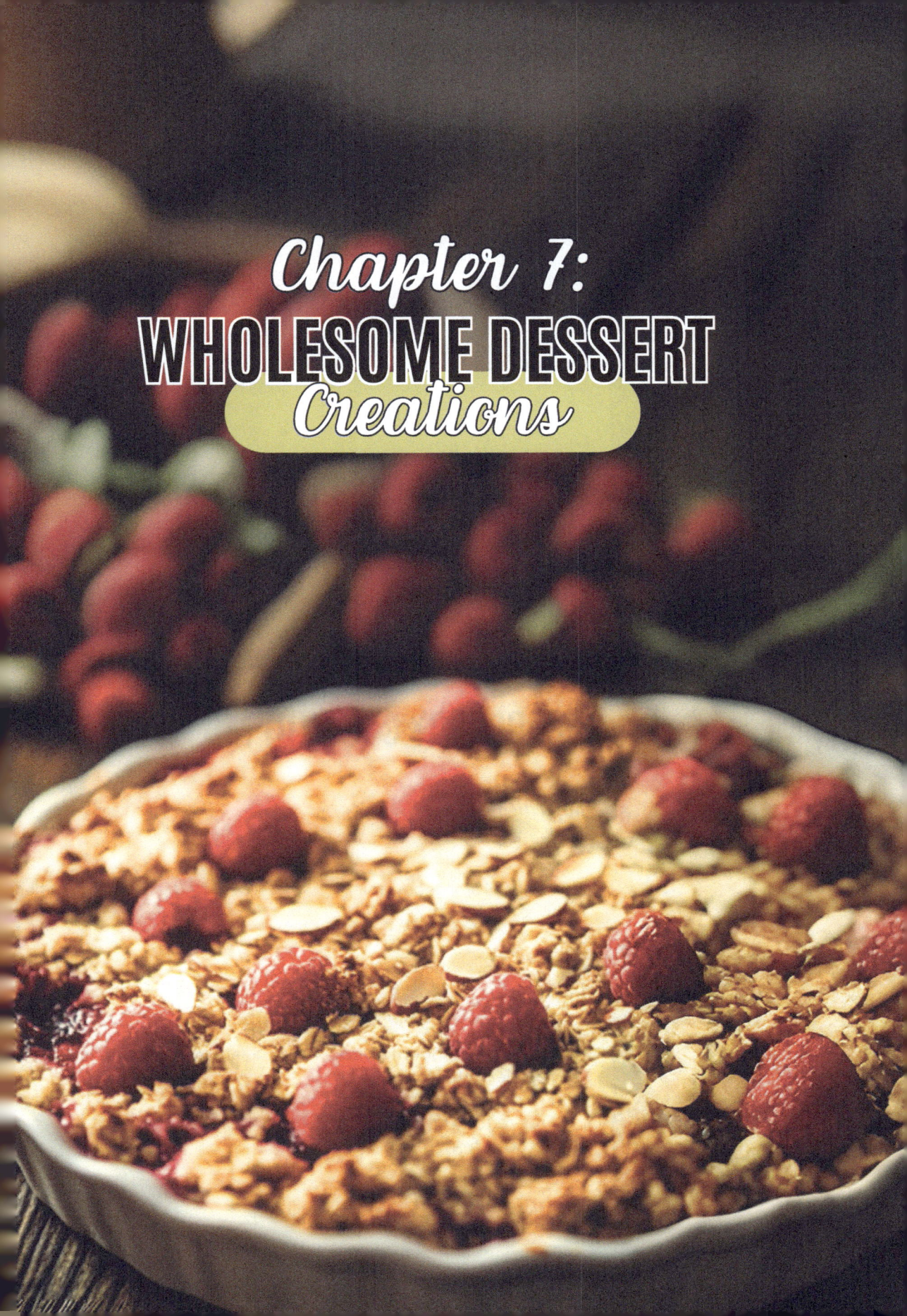

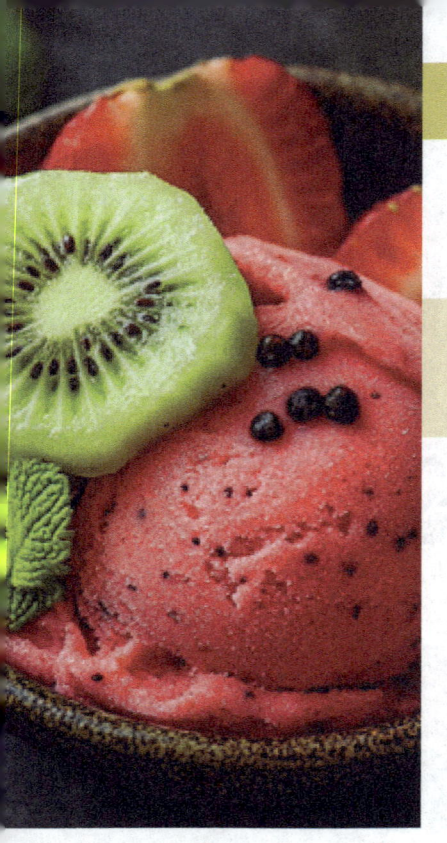

STRAWBERRY AND KIWI SORBET

Ingredients:

- 1 cup/150g fresh strawberries, hulled
- 1 kiwi, peeled and chopped
- 1 tbsp./15ml maple syrup
- 1 tbsp./15ml fresh lemon juice

Instructions:

1. Place strawberries, kiwi, maple syrup, and lemon juice into a blender or food processor.
2. Blend until smooth, then drizzle the mixture into a shallow dish.
3. Freeze for 4 hours, stirring once or twice during freezing to ensure an even texture.
4. Scoop and serve immediately.

Easy | 2 Servings | 5 min | 4 hours freezing time

Per serving:
Calories: 170 kcal | Fat: 0g | Carbs: 31g | Protein: 1g | Fiber: 4g | Sugar: 25g

---

RASPBERRY COCONUT MILK POPSICLES

Easy | 2 Servings | 10 min | 4 hours freezing time

Ingredients:

- 1 cup/240ml coconut milk (unsweetened)
- ½ cup/75g fresh raspberries
- 1 tbsp./15ml maple syrup

Instructions:

1. Blend the raspberries, coconut milk, and maple syrup in a blender until smooth.
2. Pour the mixture into popsicle molds.
3. Freeze for 4 hours, or until solid.
4. Remove from molds and serve.

Per serving:
Calories: 170 kcal | Fat: 9g | Carbs: 13g | Protein: 1g | Fiber: 3g | Sugar: 8g

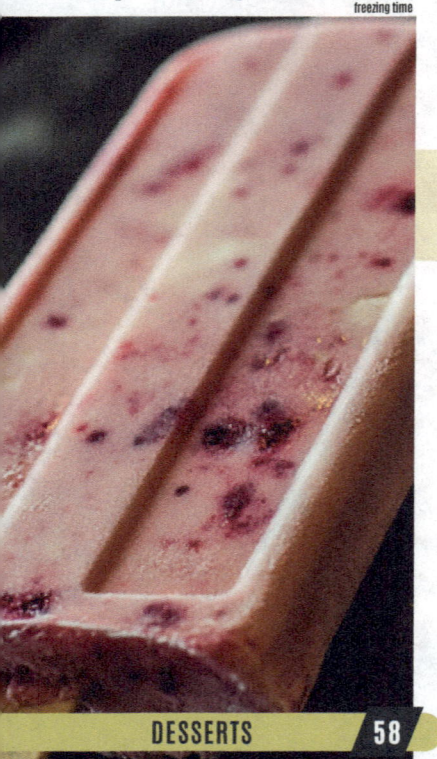

DESSERTS

KIWI AND STRAWBERRY TARTLETS

Ingredients:

- ½ cup/60g gluten-free flour
- ¼ cup/25g almond flour
- ¼ cup/60ml coconut oil, melted
- 2 tbsps./30ml maple syrup
- ¼ tsp. vanilla extract
- ¼ cup/60g coconut yogurt
- 2 kiwis, peeled and sliced
- 4 strawberries, hulled and sliced

Instructions:

1. Preheat the oven to 350°F/180°C.
2. In your bowl, mix the gluten-free flour, almond flour, melted coconut oil, maple syrup, and vanilla extract to form a dough.
3. Press the dough into mini tartlet pans and bake for 10-12 minutes until golden.
4. Let the tartlets cool completely.
5. Once cooled, fill each tartlet with coconut yogurt and top with sliced kiwi and strawberry.
6. Chill in the fridge for 30 minutes before serving.

Per serving:
Calories: 260 kcal | Fat: 15g | Carbs: 22g | Protein: 3g | Fiber: 3g | Sugar: 13g

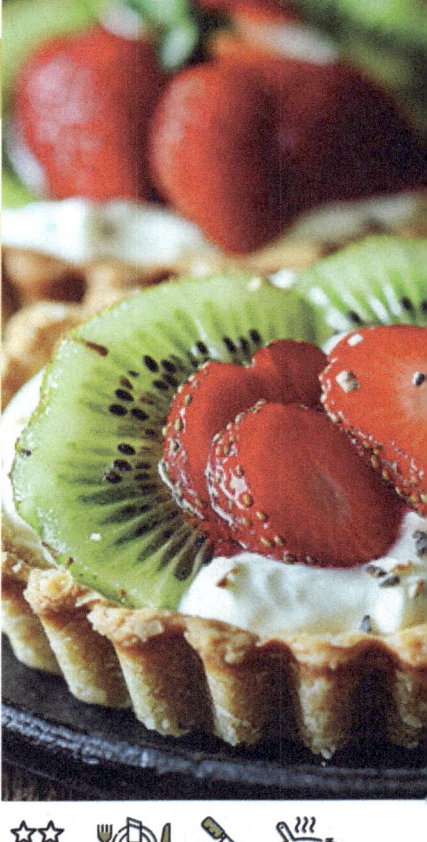

Medium 2 Servings 20 min 10-12 min

CARROT CAKE WITH ALMOND FROSTING

Medium 2 Servings 15 min 25-30 min

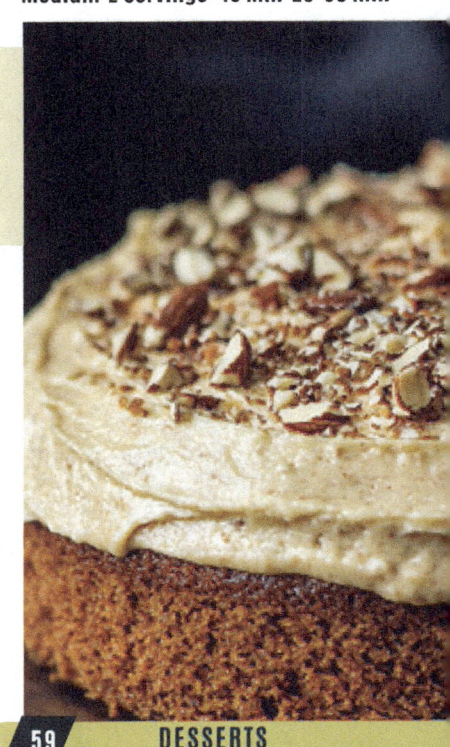

Ingredients:

- ½ cup/50g almond flour
- ½ cup/60g grated carrot
- ¼ cup/60ml maple syrup
- ¼ cup/60ml coconut oil, melted
- ¼ tsp. baking soda
- ¼ tsp. ground cinnamon
- ¼ tsp. vanilla extract

For the Frosting:
- ¼ cup/60g almond butter
- 2 tbsps. coconut oil, melted
- 1 tbsp./15ml maple syrup

Instructions:

1. Preheat the oven up to 350°F/180°C then lightly grease a small baking pan. In a bowl, mix grated carrot, almond flour, maple syrup, melted coconut oil, baking soda, cinnamon, and vanilla extract.
2. Place the batter into the prepared pan then bake for 25-30 minutes, or until a toothpick placed comes out clean.
3. While the cake is baking, prepare the frosting by blending almond butter, coconut oil, and maple syrup until smooth and creamy. Let the cake to cool completely before frosting with the almond butter mixture. Serve and enjoy!

Per serving:
Calories: 270 kcal | Fat: 18g | Carbs: 14g | Protein: 4g | Fiber: 3g | Sugar: 9g

DESSERTS

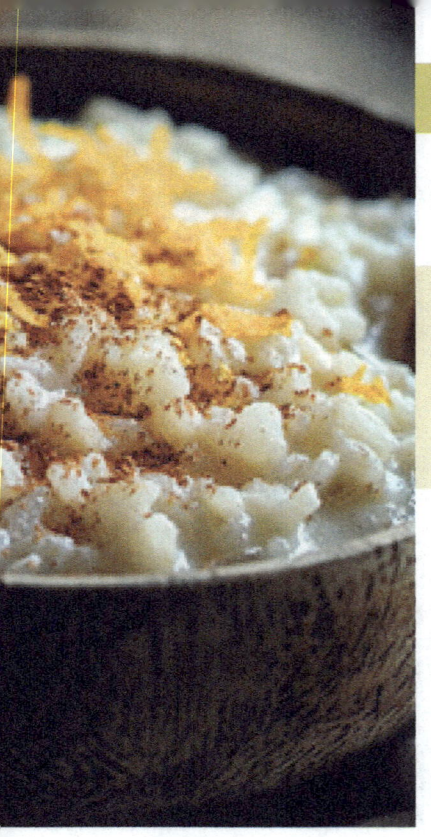

COCONUT RICE PUDDING WITH ORANGE

Ingredients:

- ½ cup/90g cooked white rice
- ½ cup/120ml coconut milk (unsweetened)
- ¼ cup/60ml almond milk
- 1 tbsp./15ml maple syrup
- ¼ tsp. ground cinnamon
- Zest of ½ orange
- 1 tbsp./15ml fresh orange juice

Instructions:

1. In a saucepan, combine the rice, almond milk, maple syrup, and cinnamon.
2. Bring to a simmer set to medium heat then cook, stirring occasionally, for 15-20 minutes, until thickened.
3. Remove from heat then stir in the orange zest and juice.
4. Serve warm or chilled.

Easy | 2 Servings | 10 min | 0 min

Per serving:
Calories: 270 kcal | Fat: 12g | Carbs: 28g | Protein: 2g | Fiber: 1g | Sugar: 12g

Easy | 2 Servings | 10 min | 25-30 min

RASPBERRY AND ALMOND CRUMBLE

Ingredients:

- ½ cup/50g almond flour
- ¼ cup/20g gluten-free oats
- 2 tbsps./30ml maple syrup
- 1 tbsp. coconut oil, melted
- ¼ tsp. ground cinnamon
- ½ cup/60g fresh raspberries
- 10 pcs/12g sliced almonds

Instructions:

- Preheat the oven up to 350°F/180°C then grease a small baking dish.
- In your bowl, combine almond flour, oats, maple syrup, coconut oil, and cinnamon.
- Gently mix in the raspberries and place the mixture into the baking dish.
- Sprinkle sliced almonds on top.
- Bake for 25-30 minutes until golden and bubbling.
- Let cool before serving.

Per serving:
Calories: 250 kcal | Fat: 15g | Carbs: 16g | Protein: 4g | Fiber: 5g | Sugar: 8g

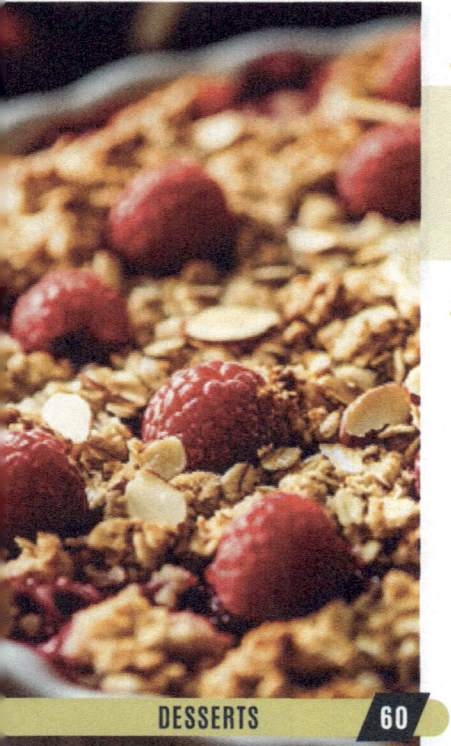

DESSERTS

RICE PUDDING

Ingredients:

- 2 cups/480ml lactose-free milk
- ½ cup/100g rice (arborio, white, or basmati)
- 1 tbsp. sugar
- Topping suggestions: ground cinnamon, walnuts, maple syrup, grated dark chocolate, blueberries, strawberries, banana, passionfruit

Instructions:

1. Pour the lactose-free milk into a medium saucepan.
2. Set the saucepan over medium heat and warm the milk until it's nearly boiling. Lower the heat, add the rice, and let it simmer.
3. Stir in 1 tbsp./15g of sugar and stir frequently. Let the mixture cook for about 20 minutes, or until the rice is tender then the pudding has thickened to your preference. If it becomes too thick, place more milk; if it's too thin, continue cooking until it thickens. Stir regularly to avoid burning the milk or rice sticking to the bottom of the pan. Once the pudding is cooked, remove it from the heat and serve.
4. Enjoy the pudding hot or cold, topped with your favorite ingredients, such as cinnamon, grated dark chocolate, maple syrup, or fresh fruit. For added flavor, you can also stir in orange or lemon zest while cooking.

Per serving:
Calories: 326kcal | Fat: 9g | Carbs: 40g | Protein: 10g | Fiber: 0g | Sugar: 20g

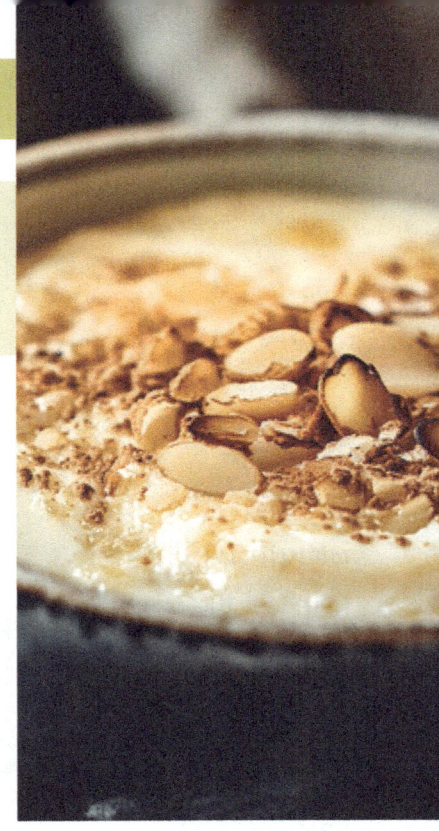

Medium | 2 Servings | 5 min | 30 min

COCONUT MACAROONS

Medium | 2 Servings | 10 min | 12-15 min

Ingredients:

- 1 ½ cups/120g shredded coconut (unsweetened)
- 2 tbsps./30ml maple syrup
- ¼ cup/60ml egg whites (from 2 large eggs)
- ½ tsp. vanilla extract

Instructions:

1. Preheat the oven up to 350°F/180°C then line a baking sheet using parchment paper.
2. Using a mixing bowl, whisk the egg whites until they form stiff peaks.
3. Gently fold in the shredded coconut, maple syrup, and vanilla extract.
4. Scoop spoonsful of the mixture and place them onto the prepared baking sheet.
5. Bake for 12-15 minutes, or until golden brown.
6. Allow to cool before serving.

Per serving:
Calories: 200 kcal | Fat: 11g | Carbs: 14g | Protein: 2g | Fiber: 2g | Sugar: 7g

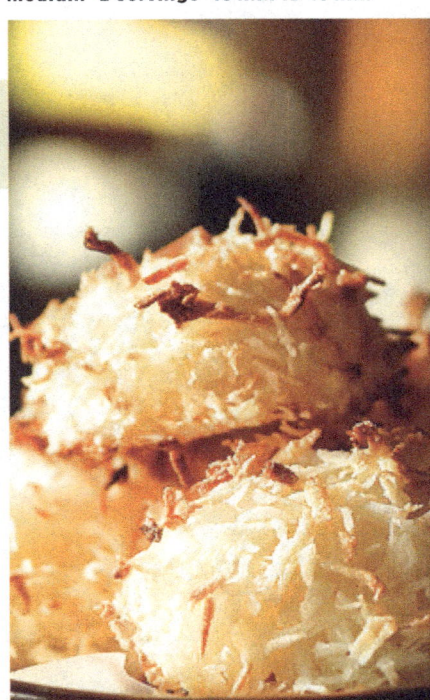

DESSERTS

WATTLESEED SELF-SAUCING PUDDING

Medium | 2 Servings | 25 min | 45 min

Ingredients:

- 2 tbsps. /8g wattleseeds (or 1-2 tbsp instant coffee)
- ½ cup/60g gluten-free flour
- ⅓ cup/67g caster sugar
- ¼ cup/25g cocoa powder
- 1 tbsp. olive oil
- ½ cup/60g spinach, chopped
- ¼ cup/30g pumpkin seeds
- Salt and pepper to taste

Instructions:

1. Preheat the oven to 350°F/180°C and prepare a baking dish or 2 ramekins by greasing with oil or butter. Soak wattleseeds in boiling water for 20 minutes and then drain.
2. In a medium-size bowl, combine the gluten-free flour, caster sugar, and 2 tablespoons/25g cocoa powder. Stir in the low-FODMAP milk, vanilla, wattleseeds (or coffee), and melted butter. Mix until smooth. Pour into the prepared baking dish or divide between ramekins.
3. In a small bowl, mix the remaining cocoa and brown sugar. Sift this mixture over the top of the pudding batter. Then, carefully pour the boiling water over it.
4. Bake for 30-35 minutes or until the top is firm. Let it stand for about 10 minutes before serving.
5. Dust with cocoa powder and serve immediately.

Per serving:
Calories: 359 kcal | Fat: 5g | Carbs: 60g | Protein: 3g | Fiber: 4g | Sugar: 40g

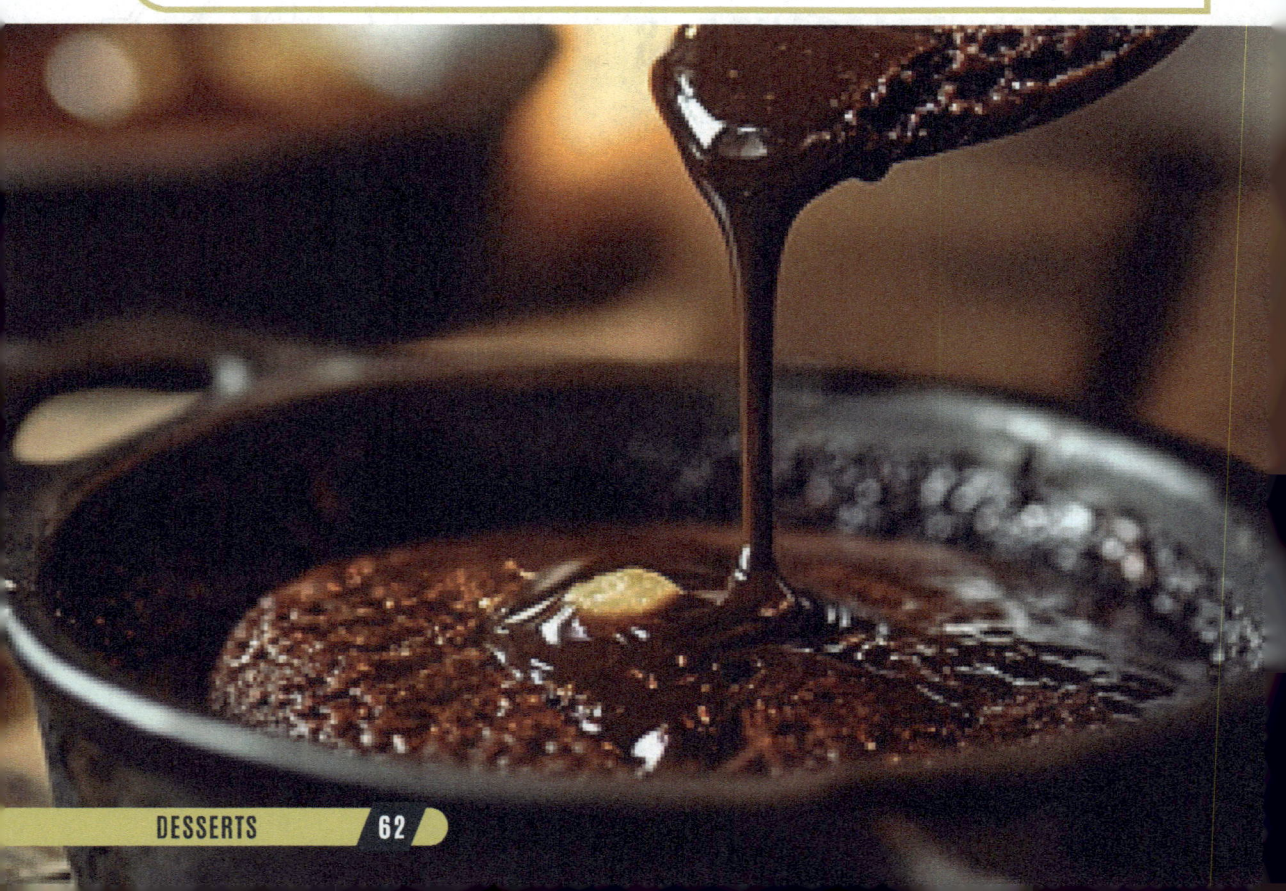

STEWED RHUBARB WITH GINGER

Ingredients:

- 2 cups/300g rhubarb, trimmed and cut into 3-inch/7.5 cm lengths
- 2 tbsps./30g brown sugar
- ¼ cup/60ml navel orange juice
- 1 tbsp. fresh ginger, peeled and finely shredded

Instructions:

1. Combine the rhubarb, orange juice, ginger, and brown sugar in a large saucepan set to medium heat.
2. Cover then bring to a simmer, cooking for 5-8 minutes, stirring occasionally, until the rhubarb softens.
3. Serve warm with your favorite cereal, like porridge, or enjoy it as a delicious and healthy dessert.

Per serving:
Calories: 238 kcal | Fat: 14g | Carbs: 9g | Protein: 4g | Fiber: 3g | Sugar: 5g

Easy | 2 Servings | 5 min | 20 min

REFRESHING MIXED FRUIT SALAD

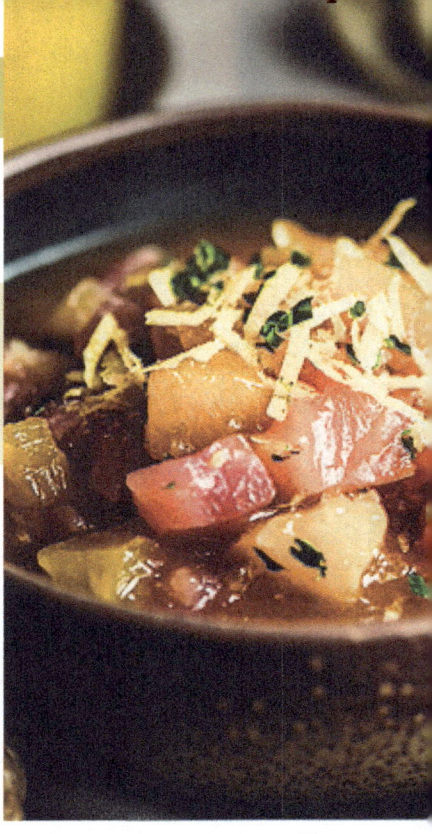

Easy | 2 Servings | 10 min | 0 min

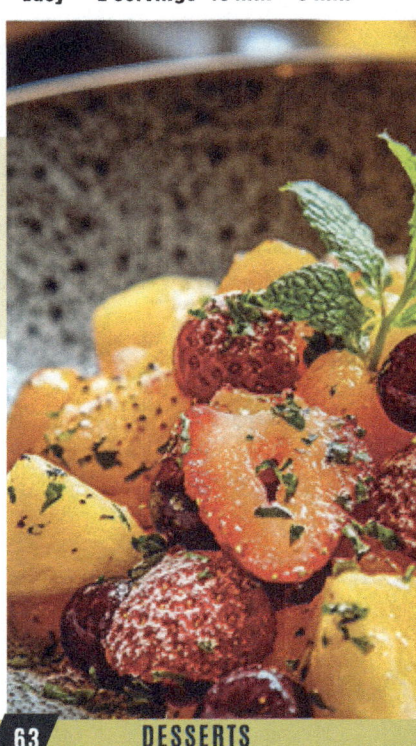

Ingredients:

- ½ cup/75g strawberries, chopped
- ½ cup/75g pineapple, chopped
- ½ cup/75g grapes, halved
- ½ cup/75g orange slices, chopped
- 1 tbsp. fresh mint, chopped
- 1 tsp./5ml lemon juice

Instructions:

1. Combine all the chopped fruit in a large bowl.
2. Drizzle with lemon juice then sprinkle with fresh mint.
3. Toss gently and serve chilled.

Per serving:
Calories: 150 kcal | Fat: 0g | Carbs: 26g | Protein: 1g | Fiber: 3g | Sugar: 22g

DESSERTS

LEMON MYRTLE SORBET

Ingredients:

- 1¾ cups/420ml water
- 1 cup/200g caster sugar
- 1⅔ cups/400ml freshly squeezed lemon juice
- Zest of 1 lemon
- ⅓ cup/80ml freshly squeezed lime juice
- Zest of 1 lime
- 1 tsp. ground lemon myrtle leaf

Instructions:

1. In a medium saucepan, combine the water and caster sugar. Stir set to medium heat until the sugar dissolves. Let the mixture cool completely.
2. Stir in the lemon juice, lime juice, lemon zest, lime zest, and ground lemon myrtle until well combined.
3. Pour the mixture into a freezer box or a large plastic container. Freeze for about 1.5 hours.
4. After 1.5 hours, break up the ice crystals using electric beaters, a fork, or a whisk. Repeat the process every hour for 4 hours or until the sorbet is firm but still easy to scoop.
5. Once the sorbet has reached the desired consistency, it is ready to serve.

Per serving:
Calories: 184 kcal | Fat: 0g | Carbs: 32g | Protein: 0g | Fiber: 1g | Sugar: 32g

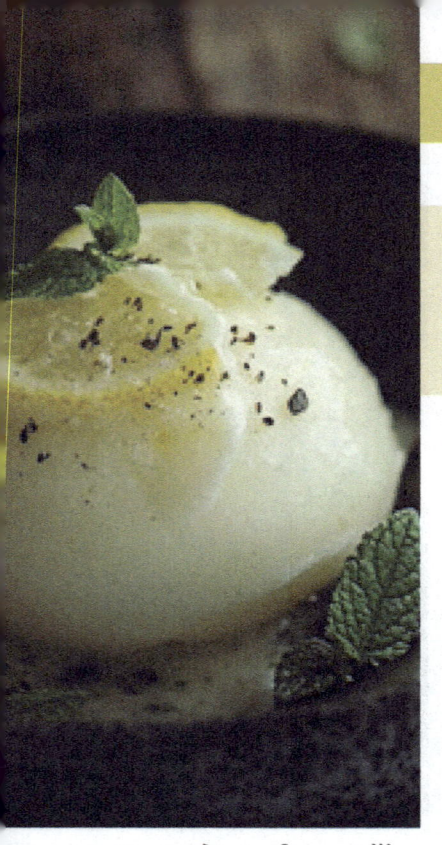

Medium | 2 Servings | 10 min | 1.5 hours freezing time

Medium | 2 Servings | 15 min | 30-35 min

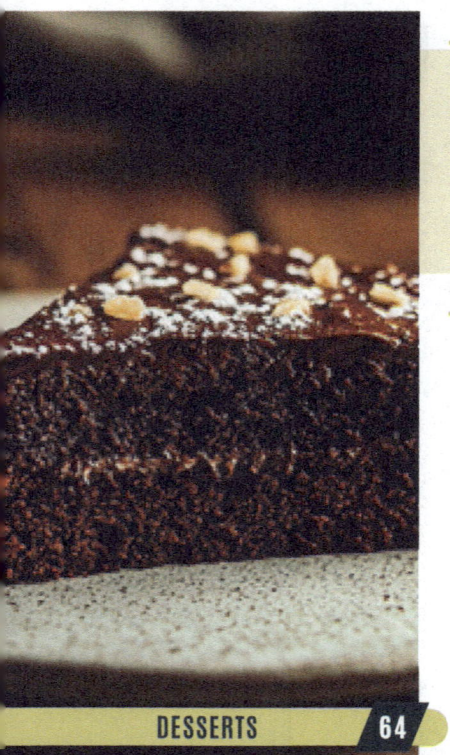

ZUCCHINI CHOCOLATE CAKE

Ingredients:

- ½ cup/60g almond flour
- ¼ cup/30g cocoa powder
- ½ cup/60g grated zucchini (excess moisture squeezed out)
- ¼ cup/60ml maple syrup
- 2 eggs
- ¼ cup/60ml coconut oil, melted
- 1 tsp./5ml vanilla extract
- ¼ tsp. baking soda
- Pinch of salt

Instructions:

1. Preheat the oven up to 350°F/180°C then lightly grease a small baking dish.
2. In a bowl, mix together cocoa powder, almond flour, and baking soda.
3. Add the zucchini, eggs, melted coconut oil, maple syrup, and vanilla extract, then stir to combine.
4. Place the batter into the prepared dish and bake for 30-35 minutes, or until a toothpick placed comes out clean.
5. Allow to cool before serving.

Per serving:
Calories: 290 kcal | Fat: 18g | Carbs: 22g | Protein: 6g | Fiber: 4g | Sugar: 12g

DESSERTS

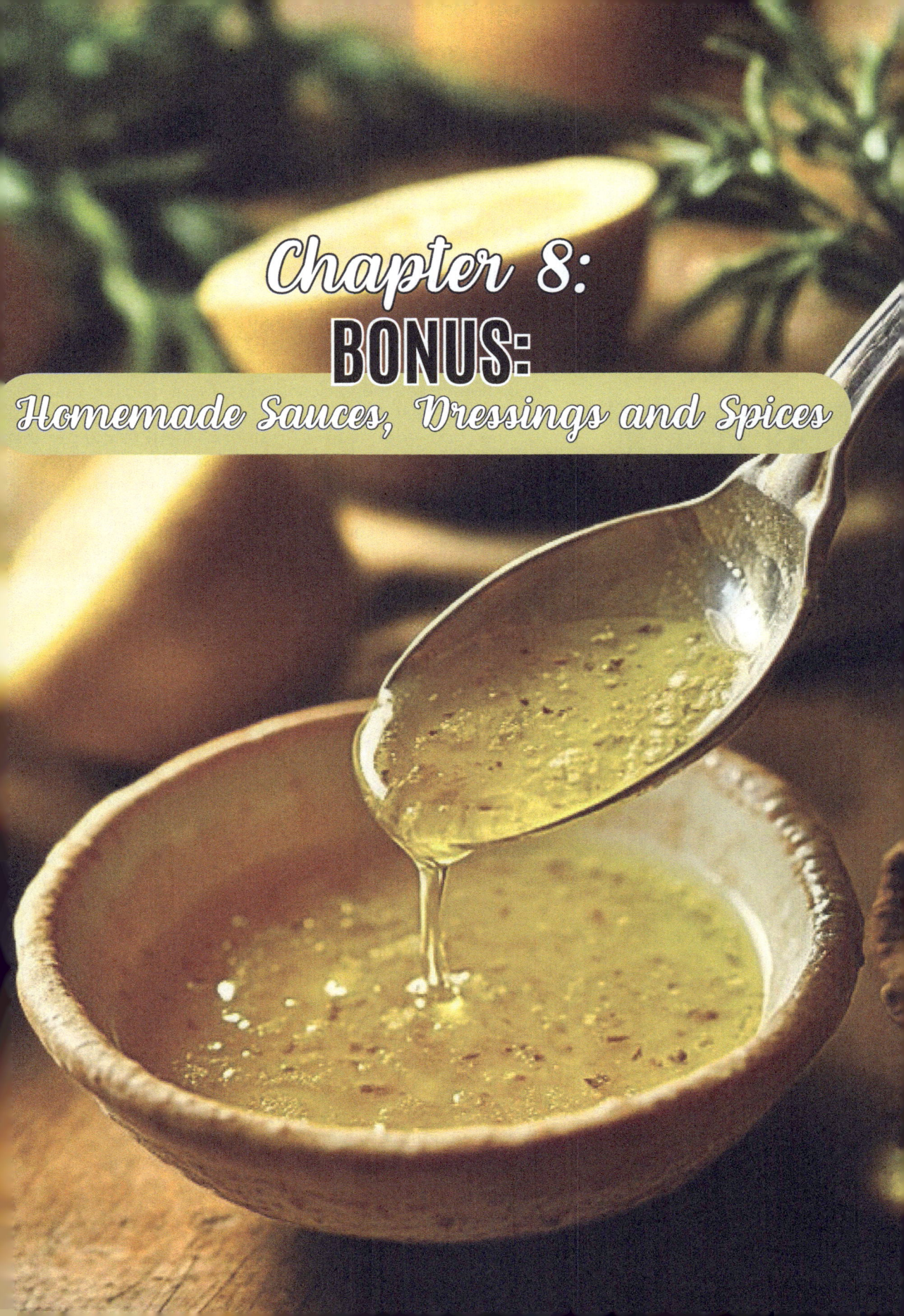

Chapter 8:
BONUS:
Homemade Sauces, Dressings and Spices

HOMEMADE TOMATO SAUCE

Ingredients: **Yield:** 2 cups/480ml

- 4 large ripe tomatoes or 1 can (400g) diced tomatoes (no added garlic or onion)
- 1 tbsp. Garlic-Infused Olive Oil (see recipe p.70)
- 1 tsp. dried oregano
- 1 tsp. dried basil
- ½ tsp. salt (optional)
- ¼ tsp. black pepper
- 1 tbsp. fresh parsley, chopped (optional)
- 1 tsp. sugar (optional, to balance acidity)

Instructions:

1. If using fresh tomatoes, score the bottoms with an "X" and blanch them in boiling water for 1-2 minutes. Remove the skins and chop them. If using canned tomatoes, simply drain and chop them. Heat the garlic-infused oil in a medium saucepan over medium heat.
2. Add the chopped tomatoes (fresh or canned) to the pan then simmer for 20-25 minutes, stirring occasionally.
3. Stir in oregano, basil, salt, pepper, and sugar (if using). Continue cooking for another 5 minutes.
4. Once the sauce reaches your desired thickness, remove from heat. Blend with an immersion blender for a smoother sauce, if desired. Stir in fresh parsley if using and let the sauce cool before storing.

per ¼ cup/60ml
Calories: 25 kcal | Fat: 2g | Carbs: 5g | Protein: 1g | Fiber: 1g | Sugar: 1g

Easy | 2 Servings | 10 min | 30 min

HOMEMADE TAHINI

Ingredients: **Yield:** 1 cup/240ml

- 1 cup/150g sesame seeds (hulled)
- ½ tsp. salt (optional)
- 2-3 tbsps. olive oil (or another neutral oil)

Instructions:

1. Toast the sesame seeds in a dry pan set to medium heat for about 5 minutes, stirring frequently until golden brown. Be careful not to burn them.
2. Once toasted, remove the sesame seeds from the pan and let them cool for a few minutes.
3. Place the sesame seeds to a food processor or blender. Blend for about 1-2 minutes until the seeds begin to break down.
4. Add the olive oil 1 tablespoon/15ml at a time and continue blending until the tahini reaches a smooth and creamy consistency. If it's too thick, add a little more oil.
5. Stir in salt, if using, and blend again.
6. Store the tahini in an airtight container in the refrigerator for up to 2 weeks.

per tablespoon/15ml
Calories: 90 kcal | Fat: 8g | Carbs: 3g | Protein: 3g | Fiber: 0g | Sugar: 0g

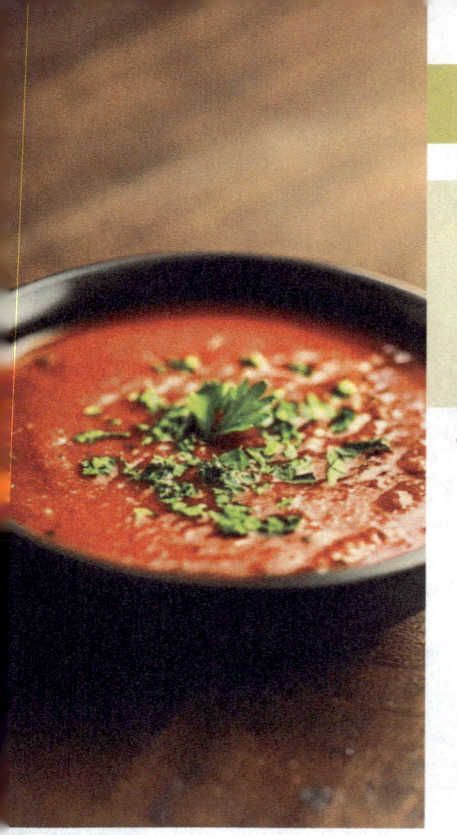

Easy | 2 Servings | 5 min | 5-10 min

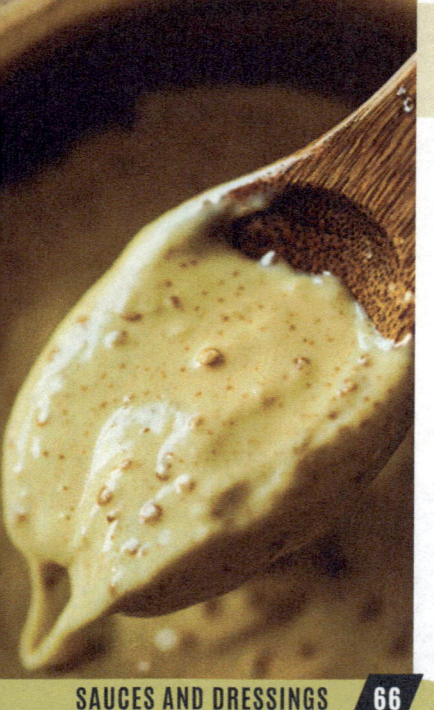

SAUCES AND DRESSINGS

HOMEMADE VEGETABLE BROTH

Ingredients:

Yield: 4 cups/960ml

- 4 cups/960ml water
- 1 medium carrot, peeled and chopped
- 2 celery stalks, chopped
- 1 small zucchini, chopped
- 1 small potato, peeled and chopped
- 1 bay leaf
- 1 tsp. black peppercorns
- 1 tbsp. fresh parsley, chopped
- 1 tsp. dried thyme (optional)
- 1 small bunch of green leek leaves (chopped, green parts only)
- 2–3 fresh sprigs of thyme or rosemary (optional)

Instructions:

1. Place the water, carrot, celery, zucchini, potato, bay leaf, black peppercorns, green leek leaves, and herbs (if using) into a medium pot.
2. Bring the mixture to a boil set to medium-high heat.
3. Once boiling, reduce the heat to a simmer then cook uncovered for 45 minutes to 1 hour, stirring occasionally.
4. After cooking, remove the pot from the heat then strain the broth through a fine-mesh sieve into a clean bowl or container, discarding the solids.
5. Stir in fresh parsley and let the broth cool. Season using a pinch of salt if desired.

per cup/240ml
Calories: 15 kcal | Fat: 0g | Carbs: 3g | Protein: 1g | Fiber: 1g | Sugar: 1g

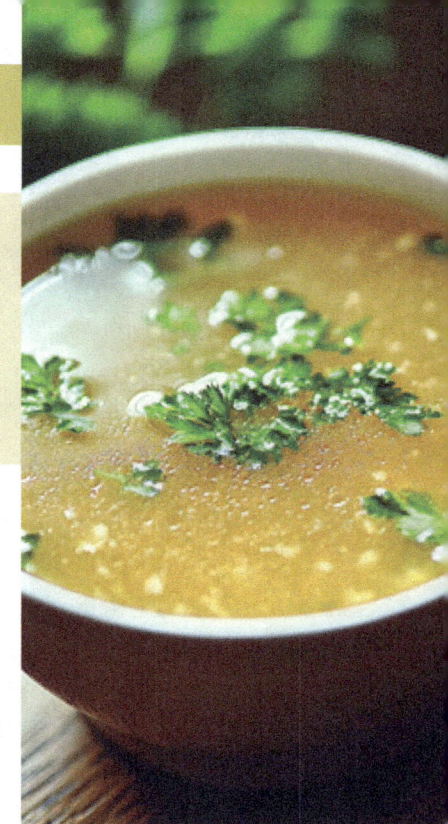

Easy | 2 Servings | 10 min | 1 hour

FRESH HERB PESTO SAUCE

Ingredients:

Yield: ¾ cup/180ml

- ½ cup/24g fresh basil leaves
- ¼ cup/12g fresh parsley leaves
- ¼ cup/30g pine nuts (or walnuts)
- ¼ cup/60ml extra virgin olive oil
- 2 tbsps./10g grated Parmesan (or dairy-free alternative)
- 1 tbsp./15ml lemon juice
- Salt to taste

Instructions:

1. In a food processor, combine basil, parsley, pine nuts, and Parmesan.
2. Pulse until the herbs are finely chopped.
3. With the processor running, slowly drizzle olive oil until the pesto reaches a thick consistency.
4. Place lemon juice and salt, and pulse to combine.
5. Serve with pasta, grilled vegetables, or meats. Store in the fridge for up to 1 week.

per ¾ cup/180ml
Calories: 230kcal | Fat: 17g | Carbs: 3g | Protein: 4g | Fiber: 1g | Sugar: 1g

Medium | 2 Servings | 10 min | 0 min

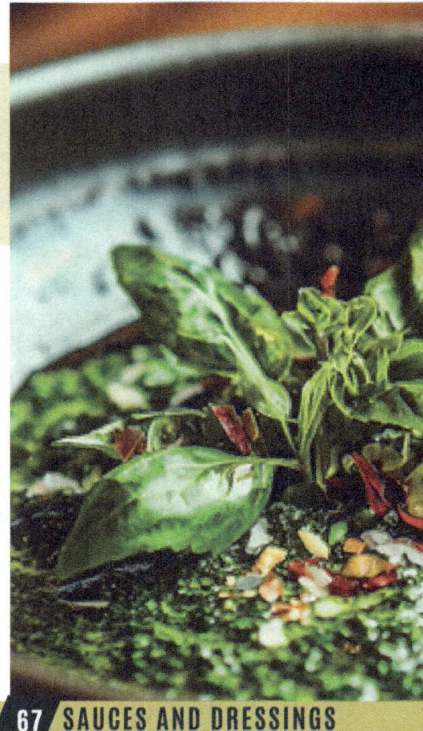

SAUCES AND DRESSINGS

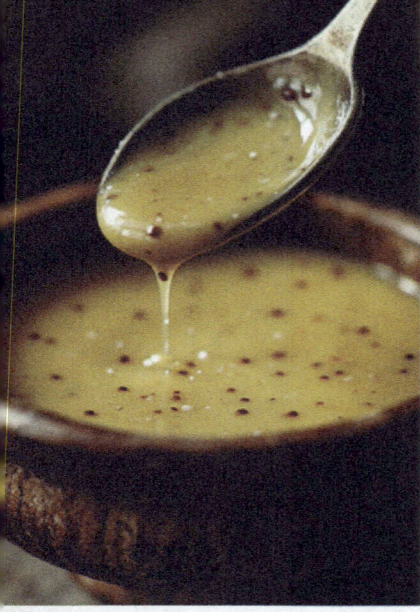

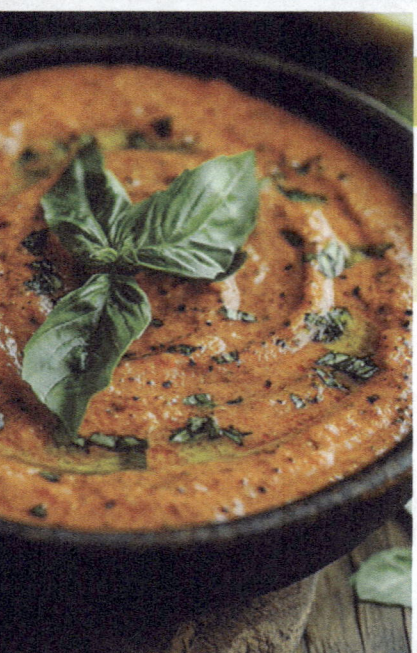

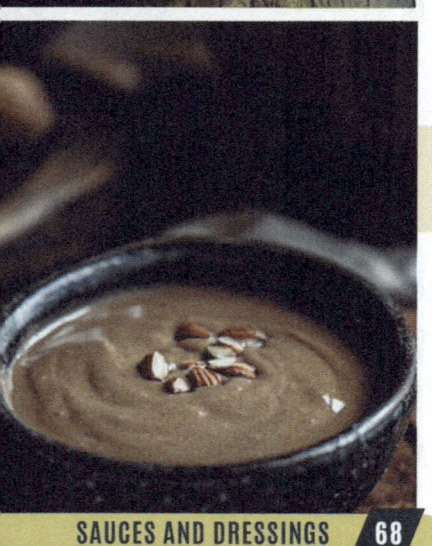

SWEET MUSTARD SAUCE

Ingredients: Easy | 2 Servings | 5 min | 0 min — **Yield:** ¼ cup/60ml

- 2 tbsps./30ml Dijon mustard
- 1 tbsp./15ml maple syrup
- 1 tbsp./15ml apple cider vinegar
- Pinch of salt

Instructions:

1. Whisk together Dijon mustard, apple cider vinegar, maple syrup, and salt in a small bowl until smooth.
2. Serve immediately or refrigerate for up to a week.
3. Use as a dressing or drizzle over grilled meats or roasted vegetables.

Per tablespoon 15ml
Calories: 95 kcal | Fat: 0g | Carbs: 11g | Protein: 1g | Fiber: 0g | Sugar: 10g

ROASTED BELL PEPPER SAUCE

Ingredients: Medium | 2 Servings | 10 min | 20 min — **Yield:** 1¼ cup/360ml

- 2 green bell peppers, roasted and peeled
- 1 tbsp. olive oil
- 1 tsp./5ml lemon juice
- Salt and pepper, to taste
- 1 tbsp. fresh basil, chopped

Instructions:

1. Bring the bell peppers under a broiler or on a grill and roast until the skin blisters and chars.
2. Once roasted, peel off the skin, discard the seeds, and chop the peppers. Blend the roasted peppers, salt, olive oil, lemon juice, and pepper in a blender until smooth.
3. Stir in the chopped basil then serve over grilled chicken or vegetables.

Per tablespoon 15ml
Calories: 100 kcal | Fat: 4g | Carbs: 8g | Protein: 1g | Fiber: 2g | Sugar: 5g

ALMOND BUTTER SAUCE

Ingredients: Easy | 2 Servings | 5 min | 0 min — **Yield:** ¼ cup/60ml

- 2 tbsps./32g almond butter
- 1 tbsp./15ml water (to thin)
- 1 tsp./5ml rice vinegar
- 1 tsp./5ml maple syrup
- Pinch of salt

Instructions:

1. In a small bowl, combine water, almond butter, rice vinegar, maple syrup, and salt.
2. Whisk until smooth. Add more water for desired consistency.
3. Drizzle over roasted vegetables, grilled meats, or use as a salad dressing.

Per tablespoon 15ml
Calories: 180 kcal | Fat: 11g | Carbs: 5g | Protein: 3g | Fiber: 1g | Sugar: 2g

SAUCES AND DRESSINGS

GARLIC-INFUSED MAYO DIPPING SAUCE

Easy | 2 Servings | 5min | 0 min | **Yield:** ½ cup/120ml

Ingredients:
- ½ cup/120g mayonnaise
- 1 tbsp. Garlic-Infused Olive Oil (see recipe p.70)
- 1 tsp./5g Dijon mustard
- 1 tsp./5ml lemon juice
- ¼ tsp. salt
- ¼ tsp. black pepper

Instructions:
1. In a small bowl, combine the garlic-infused oil, lemon juice, mayonnaise, Dijon mustard, salt, and pepper.
2. Stir well until the mixture is smooth and fully combined.
3. Adjust seasoning to taste, adding more salt, lemon, or mustard if desired. Serve immediately with your sweet potato wedges or refrigerate for later use (store in an airtight container for up to a week).

Per tablespoon 15ml
Calories: 45 kcal | Fat: 4g | Carbs: 1g | Protein: 0g | Fiber: 0g | Fiber: 1g | Sugar: 1g

GINGER AND SOY MARINADE

Easy | 2 Servings | 5 min | 0 min | **Yield:** ¼ cup/60ml

Ingredients:
- 3 tbsps./45ml tamari soy sauce (gluten-free)
- 1 tbsp. fresh ginger, grated
- 1 tbsp./15ml rice vinegar
- 1 tsp./5ml maple syrup
- ½ tsp. sesame oil

Instructions:
1. Combine rice vinegar, tamari soy sauce, grated ginger, maple syrup, and sesame oil in a small bowl.
2. Whisk until well combined.
3. Use as a marinade for chicken, fish, or tofu, or drizzle over salads. Let marinate for at least 30 minutes before cooking.

Per tablespoon 15ml
Calories: 75 kcal | Fat: 1g | Carbs: 3g | Protein: 1g | Fiber: 0g | Sugar: 2g

LEMON VINAIGRETTE

Medium | 2 Servings | 5 min | 0 min | **Yield:** ¼ cup/60ml

Ingredients:
- 3 tbsps. extra virgin olive oil
- 1 tbsp./15ml lemon juice
- Salt, to taste
- Freshly ground black pepper, to taste

Instructions:
1. In a small bowl or jar, combine olive oil and lemon juice.
2. Add salt and pepper to taste.
3. Whisk or shake well until emulsified.
4. Serve immediately over salads or store in the fridge for up to a week.

Per tablespoon 15ml
Calories: 200 kcal | Fat: 14g | Carbs: 1g | Protein: 0g | Fiber: 0g | Sugar: 0g

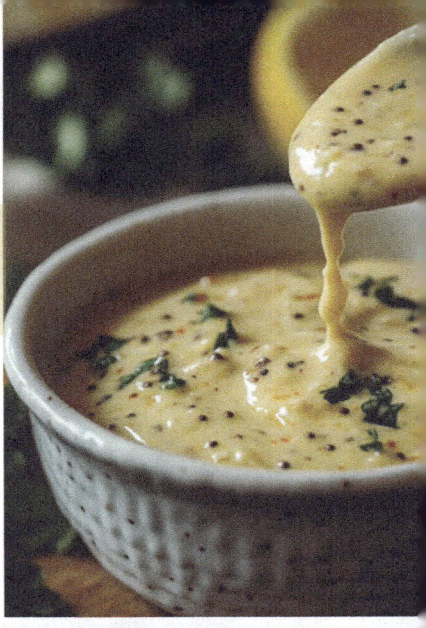

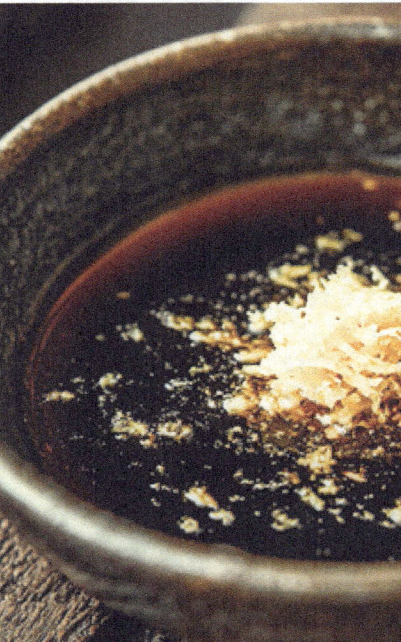

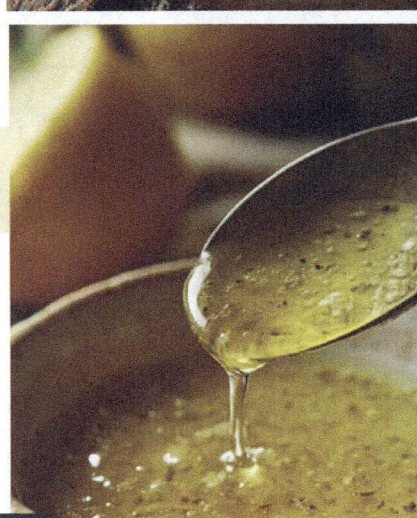

SAUCES AND DRESSINGS

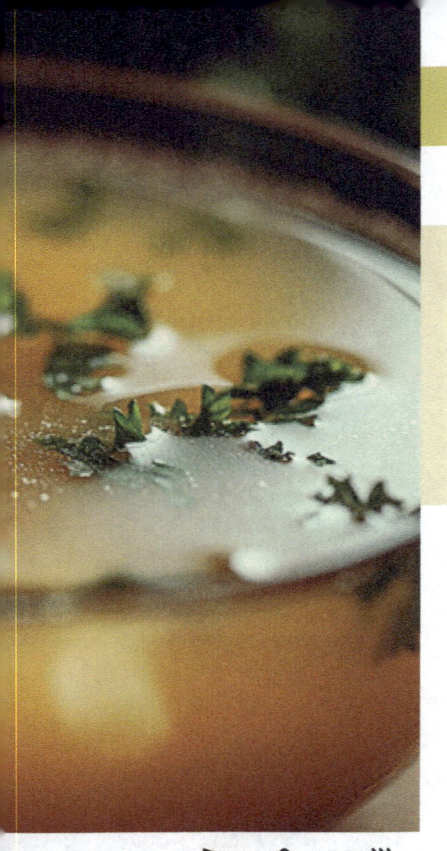

HOMEMADE CHICKEN STOCK

Ingredients:

- 4 cups/960ml water
- 1 medium carrot, chopped
- 2 celery stalks, chopped
- 1 small zucchini, chopped
- 1 small potato, peeled and chopped
- 1 bay leaf
- 1 tsp. black peppercorns
- 1 tbsp. fresh parsley, chopped
- 1 tsp. dried thyme (optional)
- 1 bunch of green leek leaves (chopped, green parts only)
- 2-3 fresh sprigs of thyme or rosemary (optional)

Instructions:

1. Place chicken bones, water, green leek leaves, carrot, bay leaf and peppercorns in a medium pot.
2. Boil, then reduce to a simmer. Cook uncovered for 2 hours skimming off any foam or impurities that rise to the surface.
3. Strain the stock through a fine-mesh sieve into a clean bowl or container, discarding solids.
4. Stir in parsley and let cool. Store in the refrigerator for up to 3 days or freeze for longer storage.

per cup/240ml
Calories: 25 kcal | Fat: 1g | Carbs: 1g | Protein: 4g | Fiber: 1g | Sugar: 1g

Easy | 2 Servings | 10 min | 2 hours

Easy | 2 Servings | 5 min | 10 min

GARLIC-INFUSED OLIVE OIL

Ingredients:

Yield: 1 cup

- 3 large garlic cloves (peeled, whole)
- 1 cup/240ml olive oil (extra virgin or light)

Instructions:

1. Combine the olive oil and whole garlic cloves in a small saucepan.
2. Heat the saucepan over low heat. Let the garlic gently infuse the oil for 8-10 minutes.
3. Avoid letting the oil boil or the garlic brown, as this can result in a bitter taste.
4. Remove the saucepan from heat then let the oil to cool completely.
5. Strain the oil to remove the garlic cloves then transfer the infused oil into a clean, airtight container.
6. Store in the refrigerator and use within 1 week.

per tablespoon/15ml
Calories: 119 kcal | Fat: 14g | Carbs: 0g | Protein: 0g | Fiber: 0g | Sugar: 0g

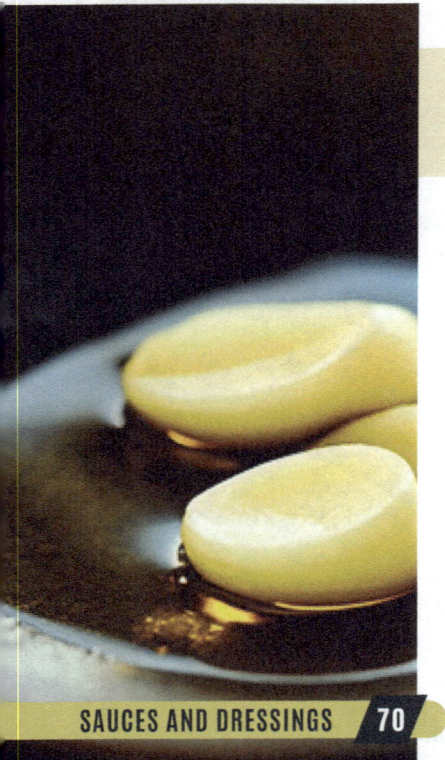

SAUCES AND DRESSINGS

Chapter 9: 28-DAY MEAL PLAN and Shopping List

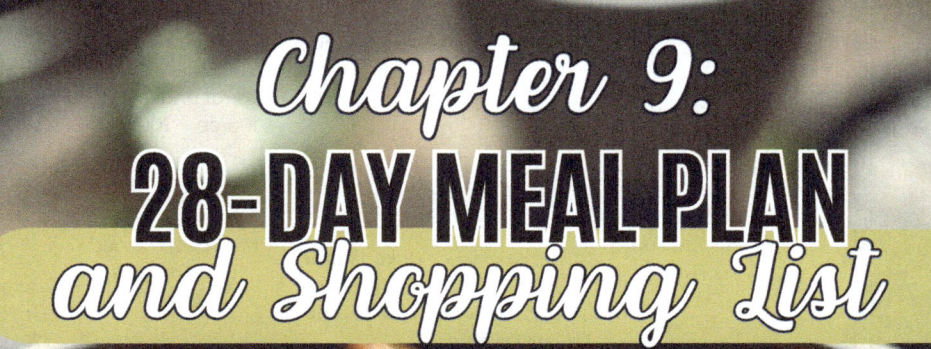

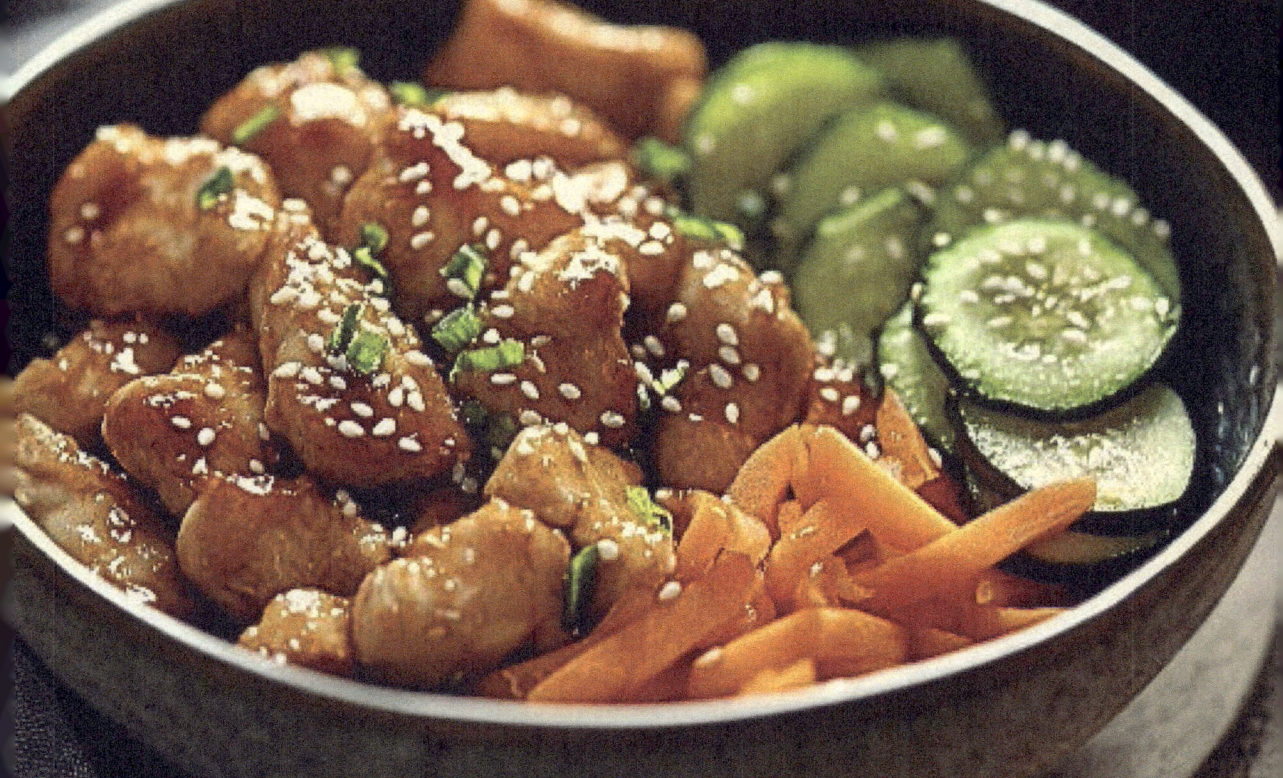

 Starting the elimination phase of the Low-FODMAP diet can feel overwhelming, especially when you're trying to figure out what to eat while avoiding high-FODMAP foods. This chapter is designed to make that process simpler and stress-free.
 Here, you'll find a thoughtfully planned 7-day meal guide tailored to kickstart your Low-FODMAP journey. Each day features breakfast, lunch, snack, dinner, and dessert to keep you satisfied and nourished without triggering discomfort. Along with delicious meal ideas, you'll also find an organized shopping list to help you stock up on everything you need for the week ahead.

Meal Plan for Elimination Week 1

Day	Breakfast	Lunch	Snack	Dinner	Dessert	Total kcal
1	Scrambled Eggs with Spinach - 230kcal	Beef Stir-Fry with Ginger and Broccoli - 370kcal Spinach and Orange Salad with Walnuts - 210kcal	Banana Energy Balls - 270kcal	Ratatouille with Eggplant and Zucchini - 230kcal Carrot and Parsnip Puree - 200kcal	Stewed Rhubarb with Ginger - 238kcal	1748
2	Quinoa Porridge with Kiwi and Pumpkin Seeds - 250kcal	Roasted Chicken Drumsticks - 370kcal Parmesan and Thyme Parsnips - 390kcal	Baked Polenta Squares - 230kcal	Moroccan Spiced Fish Tagine - 300kcal	Raspberry Coconut Milk Popsicles - 170kcal	1710
3	Fried Plantain and Fresh Mint Salad - 300kcal	Quinoa-Stuffed Bell Peppers - 320kcal	Cucumber Sticks with Hummus - 230kcal	BBQ-Style Chicken Thighs - 370kcal Spinach and Orange Salad with Walnuts - 210kcal	Rice Pudding - 326kcal	1756
4	Scrambled Eggs with Spinach - 230kcal	Beef Kebabs with Zucchini and Bell Pepper - 330kcal	Sweet Potato Chips with Coconut Oil - 240kcal	Baked Tilapia with Dill Sauce - 300kcal Sweet Potato Wedges with Rosemary - 250kcal	Stewed Rhubarb with Ginger - 238kcal	1588
5	Sweet Potato and Kale Breakfast Hash - 250kcal	Grilled Pork Tenderloin with Herbs - 350kcal	Raspberry Chia Jam - 95kcal	Sesame Chicken and Vegetable Bowl - 370kcal Maple Glazed Baby Carrots - 290kcal	Chocolate Wattleseed Self-Saucing Pudding - 359kcal	1714
6	Grilled Zucchini with Poached Eggs - 260kcal	Thai Basil Chicken Stir-Fry - 280kcal	Cucumber Sticks with Hummus - 230kcal	Sweet Potato-Crusted Chicken Tenders - 320kcal Spinach and Orange Salad with Walnuts - 210kcal	Chocolate Wattleseed Self-Saucing Pudding - 359kcal	1659
7	Tortilla Baked Eggs - 402kcal	Herb-Grilled Chicken Breast - 250kcal Zucchini and Bell Pepper Salad - 200kcal	Baked Kale Chips with Lemon Zest - 150kcal	Oven-Baked Cod with Lemon and Parsley - 230kcal Grapefruit Prawn Salad - 367kcal	Raspberry Coconut Milk Popsicles - 170kcal	1769

28-DAY MEAL PLAN

SHOPPING LIST FOR WEEK 1

PRODUCE
- 1 bag (16 oz./450g) fresh spinach
- 1 medium eggplant
- 2 zucchinis
- 4 green bell peppers
- 1 can (14.5 oz./410g) diced tomatoes
- 2 medium carrots
- 2 medium parsnips
- 1 medium sweet potato
- 1 bunch kale
- 1 bunch kale
- 2 large bell peppers
- 1 Lebanese cucumber
- 1 cucumber
- 2 medium sweet potatoes
- 1 oz./30g pumpkin seeds
- 1 lb./450g fresh strawberries
- 2 kiwis
- 1 ripe banana
- 2 ripe plantains
- 2 oranges
- ½ pink grapefruit
- 1 lemon
- 2 limes
- 1 small pineapple
- 1 small bunch (about 1 lb./450g) of grapes

NUTS AND SEEDS
- 16 oz./450g shredded coconut
- 1 bag (16 oz./450g) toasted walnuts
- 1 bag (8 oz./225g) sliced almonds
- 1 bag (8 oz./225g) roasted peanuts
- 1 bag (8 oz./225g) chia seeds

VEGETABLES
- Grains & Flours
- 1 bag (32 oz./900g) gluten-free rolled oats
- 1 bag (16 oz./450g) gluten-free flour
- 1 bag (16 oz./450g) almond flour
- 1 lb./450g polenta (cornmeal)
- 1 lb./450g hulled millet seed
- 1 box gluten-free breadcrumbs
- 6-8 gluten-free crackers

BAKING SUPPLIES
- 1 box caster sugar
- 1 bag brown sugar
- 1 bag white sugar
- 1 jar vanilla essence
- ½ cup/40g cocoa powder

DAIRY & ALTERNATIVES
- 1 dozen large eggs
- 1 carton (32 oz./950ml) lactose-free milk
- 1 pint/475ml lactose-free sour cream
- 1 container (16 oz./475g) coconut yogurt
- 1 pint cartons/475ml lactose-free heavy cream
- 8 oz./225g lactose-free cream cheese

MEAT & SEAFOOD
- 4 chicken drumsticks
- 4 chicken thighs (skin-on, bone-in)
- 4 chicken breasts (boneless, thinly sliced)
- 2 chicken breast tenders
- 2 tilapia fillets
- 2 cod fillets
- 1 pork tenderloin
- ½ lb./225g beef flank steak
- 1 lb./450g beef sirloin cubes
- ½ lb./225g peeled, cooked prawns

PANTRY STAPLES
- 1 bottle olive oil
- 1 bottle garlic-infused olive oil
- 1 bottle sesame oil
- 1 bottle rice vinegar
- 1 jar tamari (gluten-free soy sauce)
- 1 jar fish sauce
- 1 jar tahini (sesame paste)
- 1 jar almond butter
- 1 jar maple syrup
- 1 jar balsamic vinegar

SPICES & SEASONINGS
- 1 container ground cinnamon
- 1 container ground turmeric
- 1 container paprika
- 1 container smoked paprika
- 1 container ground cumin
- 1 container ground coriander
- 1 container dried basil
- 1 container dried oregano
- 1 container ground ginger
- 1 container nutmeg

HERBS
- 1 bunch fresh rosemary
- 1 bunch fresh thyme
- 1 bunch fresh dill
- 1 bunch fresh parsley
- 1 bunch fresh mint
- 1 bunch fresh basil
- 1 piece fresh ginger

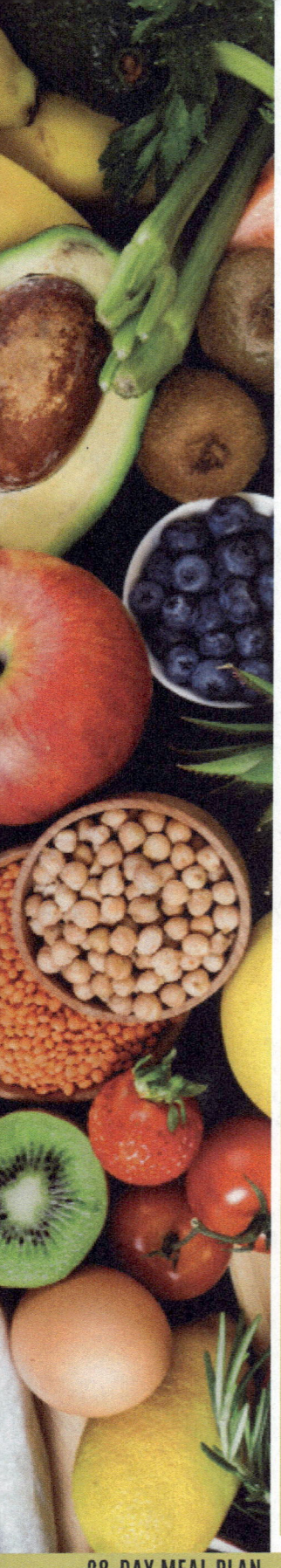

Meal Plan for Week 2

Day	Breakfast	Lunch	Snack	Dinner	Dessert	Total kcal
1	Rice Flour Crepes and Raspberries - 280kcal	Zucchini Noodles with Pesto Sauce - 300kcal Vegetable & Chickpea Soup - 230kcal	Roasted Pumpkin Seeds - 210kcal	Eggplant and Tomato Casserole - 270kcal Spaghetti Squash with Olive Oil - 200kcal	Strawberry and Kiwi Sorbet - 170kcal	1660
2	Maple Granola - 228kcal	Coconut Curry with Chicken - 450kcal Grilled Zucchini and Pepper Salad - 200kcal	Mini Zucchini Fritters - 210kcal	Garlic-Infused Shrimp Skillet - 270kcal	Carrot Cake with Almond Frosting - 270kcal	1628
3	Banana Muffins - 260kcal	Garlic-Infused Shrimp Skillet - 270kcal Sweet Potato with Rosemary - 250kcal	Roasted Chickpeas - 220kcal	Chickpea-Free Hummus Wrap - 400kcal	Raspberry Coconut Milk Popsicles - 170kcal	1570
4	Zucchini Sweet Potato Fritters - 260kcal	Tomato Basil Spaghetti Squash - 230kcal	Sweet Potato Chips - 240kcal	Baked Tilapia with Dill Sauce - 300kcal Vegetable & Chickpea Soup - 200kcal	Coconut Rice Pudding with Orange - 270kcal	1505
5	Low-FODMAP Granola with Almond Milk - 300kcal	Pan-Seared Scallops with Lemon - 230kcal	Gluten-Free Crackers with Cucumber Dill Spread - 230kcal	Roasted Vegetable Buddha Bowl - 400kcal Caprese Salad - 183kcal	Rice Pudding - 326kcal	1669
6	Pumpkin Coconut Milk Smoothie - 230kcal	Lemon and Herb Turkey Patties - 300kcal Spinach-Orange Salad with Nuts - 210kcal	Raspberry Chia Jam - 95kcal	BBQ-Style Chicken Thighs - 370kcal Beans and Carrots in Vinaigrette - 190kcal	Zucchini Chocolate Cake - 290kcal	1685
7	Coconut Rice Porridge with Cinnamon - 300kcal	Thai Basil Chicken Stir-Fry - 280kcal	Banana Energy Balls - 270kcal	Tofu Stir-Fry with Green Beans - 330kcal Baby Spinach Salad with Strawberries - 150kcal	Lemon Myrtle Sorbet - 184kcal	1514

28-DAY MEAL PLAN

SHOPPING LIST FOR WEEK 2

PRODUCE

- 2 medium zucchinis
- 2 medium sweet potatoes
- 4 medium tomatoes
- 1 small spaghetti squash
- 5-6 medium carrots
- 2 medium eggplants
- 1 green bell pepper
- 1 small head of broccoli
- 1 lb./450g Kent pumpkin
- 8 oz./225g green beans
- 8 oz./225g fresh baby spinach
- 1 medium cucumber
- 1 ripe banana
- 1 medium zucchini
- 1 medium sweet potato
- 5 oz./140g fresh raspberries
- 5 oz./140g strawberries
- 1 kiwi
- 1 lemon (for zest)
- 1 lime (for zest)
- 1 orange (for zest)

HERBS

- 1 bunch fresh basil
- 1 bunch fresh dill
- 1 bunch fresh parsley
- 1 bunch fresh rosemary
- 1 bunch fresh thyme

DAIRY AND DAIRY ALTERNATIVES

- 1 pint/475ml lactose-free milk
- 8 oz./225g lactose-free sour cream
- 4 oz./115g lactose-free cream cheese or dairy-free alternative
- 13.5 oz./400ml can coconut milk (unsweetened)
- 8 oz./225ml almond milk

GRAINS & FLOURS

- 1 lb./450g gluten-free flour
- 8 oz./225g gluten-free rolled oats
- 1 lb./450g jasmine rice
- 1 lb./450g rice flour

PROTEIN

- 2 large chicken breasts
- 4 chicken thighs
- ½ lb./225g shrimp
- 1 lb./450g ground turkey
- 8-10 large scallops

NUTS AND SEEDS

- 4 oz./115g almond flour
- 4 oz./115g raw almonds
- 2 oz./55g pumpkin seeds
- 1 oz./30g pine nuts
- 1 oz./30g chia seeds
- 0.5 oz./15g linseeds/flaxseeds
- 0.5 oz./15g sunflower seeds
- 15 oz./425g canned chickpeas (about 1 can)

OILS AND FATS

- 1 bottle olive oil
- 1 bottle garlic-infused olive oil
- 1 jar coconut oil

SWEETENERS AND SYRUPS

- 1 bottle maple syrup

SPICES AND FLAVORINGS

- 1 jar salt
- 1 jar pepper
- 1 jar paprika
- 1 jar ground cinnamon
- 1 jar ground turmeric
- 1 jar ground coriander
- 1 jar ground cardamom
- 1 jar cumin
- 1 small jar chili powder (optional)

OTHER PANTRY ITEMS

- 1 jar peanut butter, natural
- 1 jar almond butter
- 1 bottle balsamic vinegar
- 1 bottle apple cider vinegar
- 1 bottle fish sauce, gluten-free
- 1 bottle pure vanilla extract
- 1 box gluten-free crackers
- 1 pack gluten-free wraps
- 1 pack corn tortillas

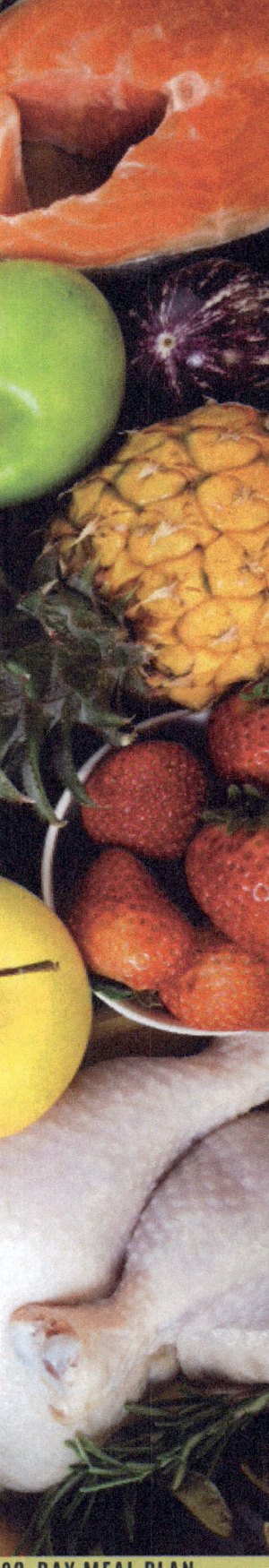

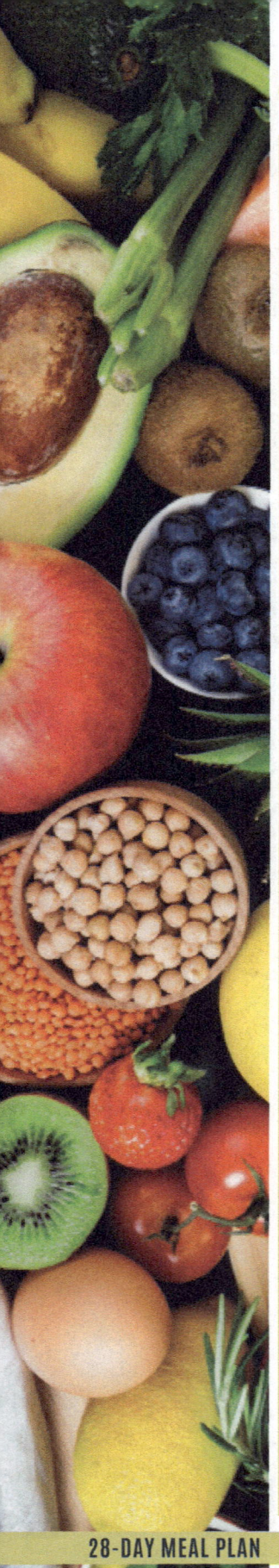

Meal Plan for Week 3

Day	Breakfast	Lunch	Snack	Dinner	Dessert	Total kcal
1	Grilled Zucchini with Poached Eggs - 260kcal	Herb-Grilled Chicken Breast - 250kcal Spaghetti Squash with Olive Oil - 200kcal	Roasted Chickpeas - 220kcal	Lentil and Spinach Curry - 350kcal Green Beans and Carrots in Lemon Vinaigrette - 190kcal	Coconut Macaroons - 200kcal	1670
2	Zucchini Sweet Potato Fritters - 260kcal	Coconut Curry with Chicken - 450kcal	Roasted Pumpkin Seeds - 210kcal	Beef with Ginger and Broccoli - 370kcal	Zucchini Chocolate Cake - 290kcal	1527
3	Cinnamon Coconut Rice Porridge - 300kcal	Moroccan Spiced Fish Tagine - 300kcal Saltbush Dukkah - 312kcal	Baked Kale Chips with Lemon Zest - 150kcal	Quinoa-Stuffed Bell Peppers - 320kcal	Coconut Rice Pudding with Orange - 270kcal	1652
4	Sweet Potato and Kale Breakfast - 250kcal	BBQ-Style Chicken Thighs - 370kcal Sweet Potato Wedges with Rosemary - 250kcal	Cucumber Sticks with Hummus - 230kcal	Lemon and Herb Turkey Patties - 300kcal Spinach Salad with Strawberries - 150kcal	Stewed Rhubarb with Ginger - 238kcal	1788
5	Banana Muffins - 260kcal	Grilled Pork with Herbs - 350kcal Quinoa Tabbouleh with Cucumber - 250kcal	Baked Polenta Squares - 230kcal	Tofu Stir-Fry with Green Beans - 330kcal	Lemon Myrtle Sorbet - 184kcal	1604
6	Scrambled Eggs with Spinach - 230kcal	Ratatouille with Eggplant - 230kcal	Mini Zucchini Fritters - 210kcal	Pan-Seared Scallops with Lemon - 230kcal Nicoise Salad with Tuna - 600kcal	Strawberry and Kiwi Sorbet - 170kcal	1670
7	Maple Granola - 228kcal	Garlic-Infused Shrimp Skillet - 270kcal Grilled Zucchini and Pepper Salad - 200kcal	Sweet Potato Chips with Coconut Oil - 240kcal	Oven-Baked Cod with Lemon - 230kcal Beans and Carrots in Vinaigrette - 190kcal	Kiwi and Strawberry Tartlets - 260kcal	1618

28-DAY MEAL PLAN

SHOPPING LIST FOR WEEK 3

PRODUCE

- 3-4 medium zucchini
- 2 lbs./900g sweet potatoes
- 1 medium cucumber
- 1 lb./450g carrots
- 1 medium eggplant
- 1 large green bell pepper
- 1 large red bell pepper
- 4-5 large kale leaves
- 1 lb./450g baby spinach
- 2-3 stalks rhubarb
- 12-15 cherry tomatoes
- 1 medium broccoli head
- 2 large kiwis
- 1 pint/340g strawberries
- 1 bunch parsley
- 1 bunch basil
- 1 bunch thyme
- 1 bunch rosemary
- 1 medium lemon
- 1 medium lime
- 1 orange

PANTRY

- 1 jar olive oil
- 1 jar garlic-infused olive oil
- 1 jar coconut oil
- 1 jar pure maple syrup
- 1 bottle balsamic vinegar
- 1 bottle apple cider vinegar
- 1 bottle tamari (gluten-free soy sauce)
- 1 jar natural peanut butter
- 1 bag (16 oz./450g) almond flour
- 1 bag (8 oz./225g) rolled oats
- 1 bag (8 oz./225g) polenta (cornmeal)
- 1 bag (16 oz./450g) Arborio rice
- 1 bag (16 oz./450g) quinoa
- 1 bag (16 oz./450g) jasmine rice

DAIRY & EGGS

- 1 dozen large eggs
- 1 small container (16 oz./475ml) lactose-free heavy cream
- 1 small container (16 oz./475g) coconut yogurt

PROTEIN

- 4 chicken thighs, skin-on, bone-in
- 1 lb./450g chicken breasts (boneless, skinless)
- 1 lb./450g ground turkey
- 2 cod fillets
- ½ lb./225g shrimp, peeled and deveined
- ½ lb./225g beef, thinly sliced (e.g., flank steak)
- 1 lb./450g pork tenderloin
- 8-10 large scallops
- 1 can tuna in oil

NUTS AND SEEDS

- 1 bag (8 oz./225g) pumpkin seeds/pepitas
- 1 bag (8 oz./225g) sesame seeds
- 1 bag (8 oz./225g) linseeds/flaxseeds
- 1 bag (8 oz./225g) chia seeds
- 1 bag (8 oz./225g) sunflower seeds
- 1 bag (8 oz./225g) buckwheat kernels
- 1 bag (8 oz./225g) macadamia nuts
- 1 bag (8 oz./225g) shredded coconut (unsweetened)

CANNED GOODS

- 1 can (15 oz./425g) coconut milk (unsweetened)
- 1 can (15 oz./425g) pumpkin puree
- 1 can (15 oz./425g) chickpeas
- 1 small can (8 oz./225g) diced tomatoes

OTHER

- 1 small jar (4 oz./115g) vanilla extract
- 1 small container (8 oz./225g) caster sugar
- 1 small jar (4 oz./115g) brown sugar
- 1 small jar (4 oz./115g) white sugar

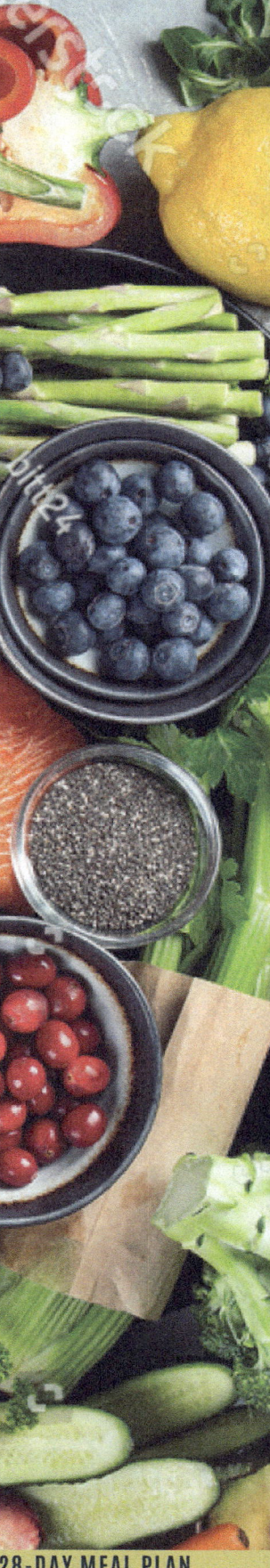

28-DAY MEAL PLAN

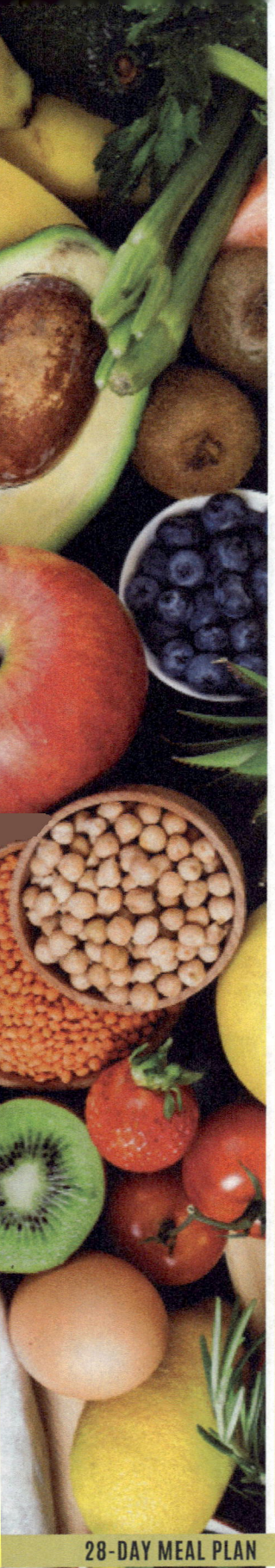

Meal Plan for Week 4

Day	Breakfast	Lunch	Snack	Dinner	Dessert	Total kcal
1	Pumpkin and Coconut Milk Smoothie - 230kcal	Quinoa-Stuffed Bell Peppers - 320kcal Grilled Zucchini and Pepper Salad - 200kcal	Baked Kale Chips with Lemon Zest - 150kcal	Zucchini Lasagna with Ricotta - 340kcal Carrot and Parsnip Puree - 200kcal	Raspberry and Almond Crumble - 250kcal	1690
2	Low-FODMAP Granola with Almond Milk - 300kcal	Beef with Ginger and Broccoli - 370kcal	Banana Energy Balls - 270kcal	Chicken with Vegetables in Sesame - 370kcal Caprese Salad - 183kcal	Carrot Cake with Almond Frosting - 270kcal	1763
3	Quinoa Porridge with Kiwi - 250kcal	Pan-Seared Scallops with Lemon - 230kcal Vegetable & Chickpea Soup - 200kca	Roasted Chickpeas - 220kcal	Shepherd's Pie with Sweet Potato - 400kcal Spaghetti Squash with Olive Oil - 200kcal	Raspberry Coconut Milk Popsicles - 170kcal	1670
4	Tortilla Baked Eggs - 402kcal	Oven-Baked Cod with Lemon - 230kcal Carrot and Parsnip Puree- 230kcal	Roasted Pumpkin Seeds - 210kcal	Grilled Pork with Herbs - 350kcal	Rice Pudding - 326kcal	1748
5	Tropical Millet Porridge - 515kcal	Zucchini Noodles with Pesto Sauce - 300kcal Saltbush Dukkah - 312kcal	Raspberry Chia Jam - 95kcal	Sweet Potato Patties- 330kcal	Refreshing Mixed Fruit Salad - 150kcal	1702
6	Rice Flour Crepes with Raspberries - 280kcal	Roasted Chicken Drumsticks - 370kcal Carrot and Parsnip Puree - 200kcal	Mini Zucchini Fritters - 210kcal	Sweet Potato-Crusted Chicken Tenders - 320kcal	Wattleseed Self-Saucing Pudding - 359kcal	1739
7	Fried Plantain and Mint Salad - 300kcal	Baked Tilapia with Dill Sauce - 300kcal Sweet Potato with Rosemary - 250kcal	Cucumber Sticks with Hummus - 230kcal	Tofu Stir-Fry with Green Beans - 330kcal	Zucchini Chocolate Cake - 290kcal	1700

28-DAY MEAL PLAN

SHOPPING LIST FOR WEEK 4

PANTRY STAPLES
- 1 jar olive oil
- 1 bottle garlic-infused olive oil
- 1 small bottle sesame oil
- 1 small bottle balsamic vinegar
- 1 small bottle rice vinegar
- 1 small bottle tamari (gluten-free soy sauce)
- 1 jar tahini (sesame paste)
- 1 lb./450g bag quinoa
- 1 lb./450g bag gluten-free rolled oats
- 1 lb./450g bag gluten-free flour
- 1 bag gluten-free breadcrumbs
- 1 lb./450g bag almond flour
- 1 jar almond butter
- 1 small jar caster sugar
- 1 small jar brown sugar
- ¼ lb./115g cocoa powder
- 1 small jar maple syrup
- 1 small jar honey
- 1 jar Dijon mustard

HERBS & SPICES
- 1 bunch fresh basil
- 1 bunch fresh parsley
- 1 bunch fresh dill
- 1 small jar dried thyme
- 1 small jar dried rosemary
- 1 small jar ground cinnamon
- 1 small jar smoked paprika
- 1 small jar ground turmeric
- 1 small jar ground cumin
- 1 small jar ground coriander
- 1 small jar ground cardamom
- small jar chili powder

DAIRY AND DAIRY ALTERNATIVES
- 1 pint/475ml lactose-free milk
- 8 oz./225g lactose-free sour cream
- 4 oz./115g lactose-free cream cheese or dairy-free alternative
- 13.5 oz./400ml can coconut milk (unsweetened)
- 8 oz./225ml almond milk

CANNED GOODS
- 1 can chickpeas
- 1 can tomato sauce (no onion or garlic)

MEAT & SEAFOOD
- 1 lb./450g pork tenderloin
- 2 chicken breasts
- 8-10 large scallops
- 2 cod fillets
- 2 tilapia fillets
- ½ lb./225g flank steak

NUTS, SEEDS & DRIED GOODS
- 1 lb./450g raw almonds
- ½ lb./225g pumpkin seeds (pepitas)
- ¼ lb./115g sunflower seeds
- ¼ lb./115g pine nuts
- ¼ lb./115g sesame seeds

VEGETABLES
- 2 lb./900g pumpkin
- 4 large zucchinis
- 4 large sweet potatoes
- 4 medium carrots
- 2 medium parsnips
- 2 cucumbers
- 1 bunch of kale
- 1 lb./450g broccoli florets
- 6 large bell peppers

MISCELLANEOUS
- 1 bottle vanilla extract
- 1 bottle lemon juice
- 1 bottle orange juice
- 1 small bag dried shredded coconut
- 1 small packet wattleseeds (or instant coffee)
- 1 pack corn tortilla

FRUITS
- 1 medium banana
- 2 medium plantains
- 1 medium kiwi
- 1 pint/300g fresh raspberries
- 1 pint/300g cherry tomatoes
- ½ lb./225g strawberries

DAIRY & ALTERNATIVES
- 1 pint/475ml almond milk
- 1 pint/475ml coconut milk
- ½ pint/240ml lactose-free milk
- ½ pint/240ml lactose-free sour cream
- ¼ pint/120ml coconut yogurt (lactose-free)

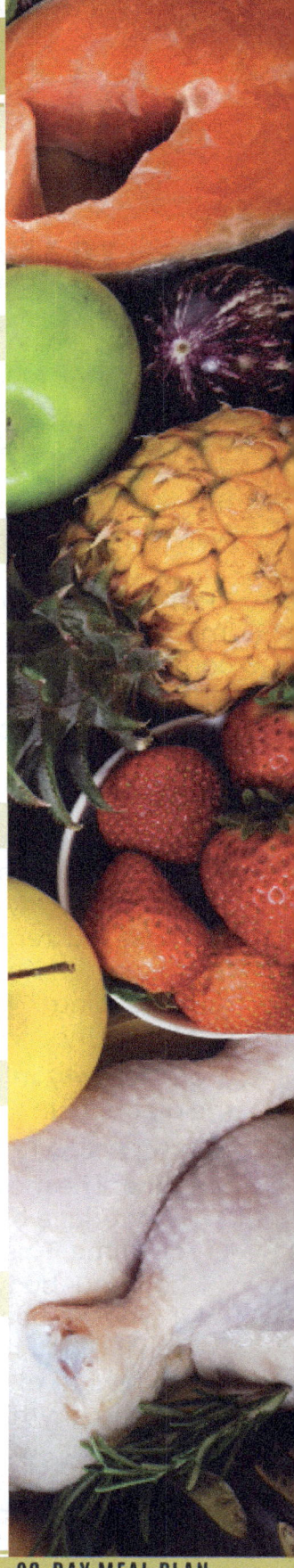

28-DAY MEAL PLAN

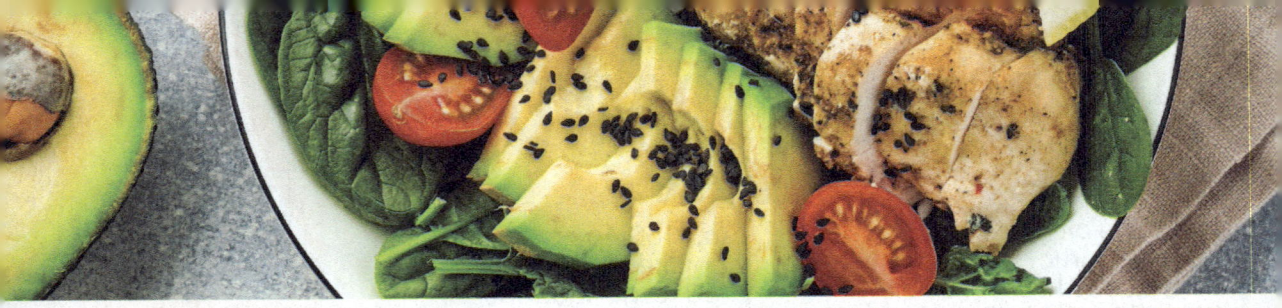

TRANSITIONING OUT OF THE DIET PHASE

After spending weeks eliminating high-FODMAP foods from your diet, you might be feeling relief from the digestive discomfort that once plagued you. But, as you approach the end of the elimination phase, you might be wondering, *What comes next?*

Transitioning out of this phase is an important step, and it's all about carefully reintroducing foods to pinpoint your triggers and gradually return to a more balanced, sustainable eating plan.

The key to transitioning out of the diet phase is patience. This isn't a race—it's a process of self-discovery. You've already made significant progress by removing high-FODMAP foods, and now, it's time to start reintroducing them slowly and strategically.

Here's how you can transition out of the diet phase:

- **Start Slowly with One Food at a Time:** The most important thing is to reintroduce one high-FODMAP food at a time. This allows you to observe how your body reacts. For example, if you've been eliminating garlic, you'll want to reintroduce it alone and wait at least 3 days before adding anything else back into your diet. This way, if any symptoms arise, you'll know exactly which food is causing the issue.
- **Monitor Symptoms:** As you reintroduce foods, be mindful of how your body responds. Take notes in a food diary to track any digestive symptoms like bloating, gas, or changes in bowel movements. It's also helpful to rate your symptoms on a scale, so you can assess how severe the reaction is.
- **Gradual Adjustments:** As you continue reintroducing foods, you may discover that some can be tolerated in small amounts, while others may be completely off-limits. The goal isn't to avoid FODMAPs forever but to find your personal tolerance level.

The goal isn't to restrict yourself forever but to find the foods that work for you.

You're working toward a personalized approach to eating that keeps your gut happy while still allowing you to enjoy a variety of foods. As you move through this phase, keep in mind that it might take time.

But with patience and awareness, you'll be able to enjoy a balanced diet without the uncomfortable symptoms you once experienced.

Are you ready to put your newfound knowledge into practice? Now that you've learned about the Low-FODMAP diet, it's time to create delicious, easy-to-make recipes!

GOOD LUCK ON YOUR DELICIOUS JOURNEY TO HEALTHIER EATING!

28-DAY MEAL PLAN

"We are what we repeatedly do. Excellence, then, is not an act, but a habit." – Aristotle

Conclusion

A BIG STEP TOWARD IMPROVING YOUR HEALTH

Wow, we've come to the end of this book! And while it might feel like a lot of information to digest (pun intended!), I want you to take a moment and give yourself credit for getting here.

Whether you're new to the Low-FODMAP diet or have been on this journey for a while, you've made a huge step toward improving your gut health and, ultimately, your overall well-being. I truly hope this book has helped demystify the process and made the Low-FODMAP diet feel like a doable, even exciting, path forward.

YOU'VE GOT THIS—NOW GO AND APPLY WHAT YOU'VE LEARNED!

The most important thing I want you to remember is that this isn't just a diet; it's a way of taking charge of your health. You've learned so much already, but the real transformation happens when you put this knowledge into action.

Start small, celebrate the wins (even the tiny ones!), and stay consistent.

If things feel overwhelming, take a deep breath. You don't have to do it all at once. Use the recipes, meal plans, and tips from this book as your foundation.

Keep referring back to the guidelines and remember that this process is all about understanding what your body needs and finding the foods that make you feel good.

This is your time to feel your best. Your gut will thank you, and so will your mind and body. I can't wait to hear how this diet helps you find balance and thrive.

SO, GO AHEAD—GET IN THE KITCHEN, EXPERIMENT WITH THOSE RECIPES, AND START MAKING POSITIVE CHANGES IN YOUR LIFE TODAY. YOU'VE GOT THIS!

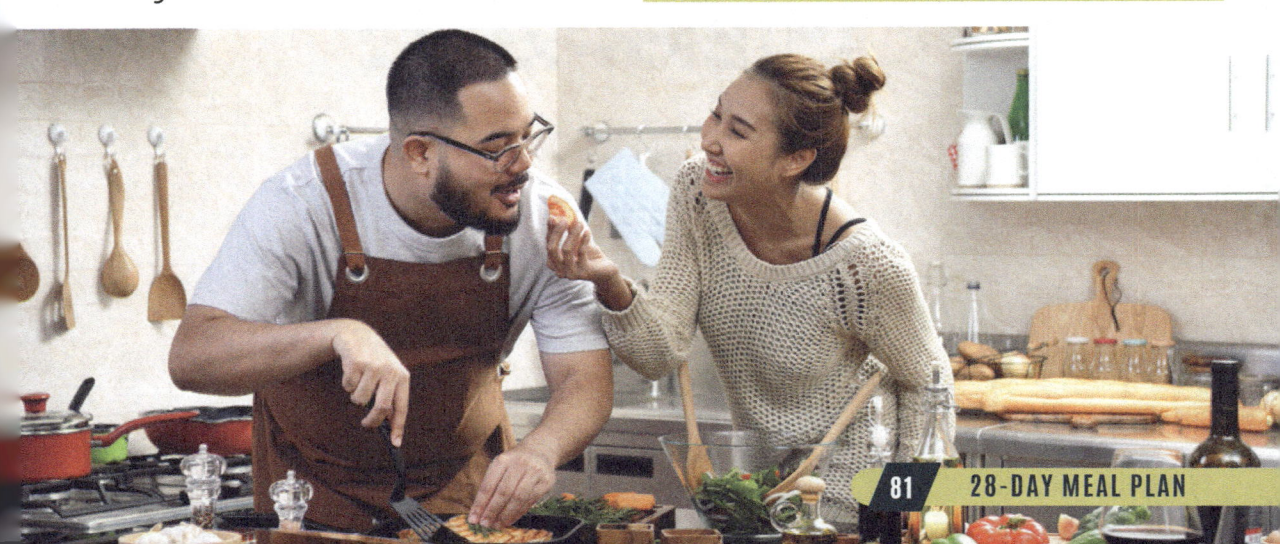

Thank You For Reading!

As an independent author with a limited marketing budget, reviews are essential for my success on Amazon platform. If you liked this book, I would be so grateful if you could share your honest thoughts!

Feel free to click the QR code below to get started! It's always a joy to hear from my readers, and I make it a point to read each and every review myself.

Made in the USA
Las Vegas, NV
23 April 2025